BEN RILEY, JAYNE HAYNES AND STEVE FIELD

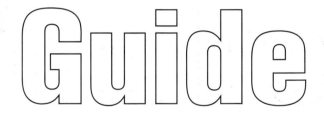

SECOND EDITION

 Royal College of
General Practitioners

The Royal College of General Practitioners was founded
in 1952 with this object:

*'To encourage, foster and maintain the highest possible standards
in general practice and for that purpose to take or join with others
in taking steps consistent with the charitable nature of that object
which may assist towards the same.'*

Among its responsibilities under its Royal Charter the
College is entitled to:

*'Diffuse information on all matters affecting general practice and
issue such publications as may assist the object of the College.'*

British Library Cataloguing-in-Publication Data
A catalogue record for this book is available from the British Library

© Royal College of General Practitioners, 2012
Published by the Royal College of General Practitioners, 2012
30 Euston Square, London NW1 2FB

Disclaimer
This publication is intended for the use of medical practitioners in the UK
and not for patients. The authors, editors and publisher have taken care to
ensure that the information contained in this book is correct to the best of their
knowledge, at the time of publication. Whilst efforts have been made to ensure
the accuracy of the information presented, particularly that related to the
prescription of drugs, the authors, editors and publisher cannot accept liability
for information that is subsequently shown to be wrong. Readers are advised
to check that the information, especially that related to drug usage, complies
with information contained in the *British National Formulary*, or equivalent,
or manufacturers' datasheets, and that it complies with the latest legislation
and standards of practice.

Designed and typeset at the Typographic Design Unit
Printed by Hobbs
Indexed by Susan Leech
ISBN 978-0-85084-339-2

The Condensed Curriculum Guide

Second Edition

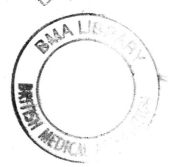
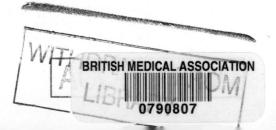

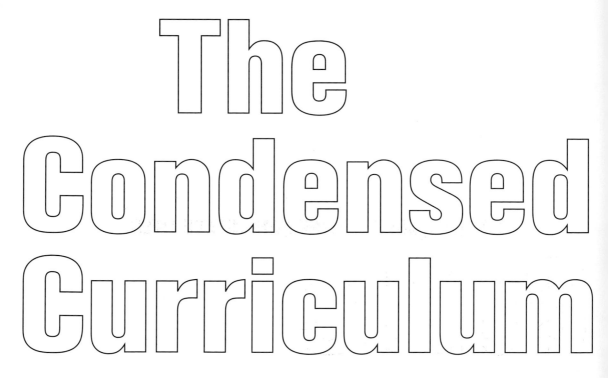

The Condensed Curriculum

FOR GP TRAINING AND THE MRCGP

To Bert, Janet, Linda, Keith, Alex and Charlotte; and to Liz, John, Richard, Harriet and Archie; who between them have given the authors nearly 300 years of unconditional support, guidance, love ... and perseverance.

Contents

About the authors   ix

Foreword to the First Edition   xi

Foreword to the Second Edition   xiii

Acknowledgements   xv

What's in this guide   xvii

Part I: The curriculum guide

1 Introducing the curriculum   3

2 Understanding the curriculum   11

3 Learning and teaching the curriculum   17

4 Succeeding at the MRCGP   37

Part II: The condensed curriculum

5 The core curriculum   77

6 The applied knowledge   131

Appendix 1:
Getting the most from specialty-based placements   303

Appendix 2:
MRCGP Consultation Observation Tool (COT)   315

Appendix 3:
Common GP topics mapped to the relevant
curriculum statements   317

Index   329

About the authors

Dr Ben Riley FRCGP is a GP in Faringdon, in rural Oxfordshire. He is the current Medical Director of Curriculum at the Royal College of General Practitioners and a member of the Postgraduate Training and Professional Development Boards. In this role, and as joint lead writer of the case to enhance and extend GP training, he is responsible for developing the framework for career-long GP education and continuing professional development. As the College's e-learning director, he oversaw the creation of hundreds of modules, courses and publications for GPs, trainees and trainers. In 2012, Ben was awarded the RCGP Certificate of Commendation for his contribution to general practice.

Dr Jayne Haynes MRCGP is a GP in a well-established training practice in the city centre of Oxford. She undertook her GP training on the Oxford Vocational Training Scheme before taking a senior registrar post in academic general practice. After working for a short spell in New Zealand, she returned to her practice in Oxford – initially as a salaried GP and now as a GP partner. She is involved in the everyday education of medical students, Foundation Year doctors and GP specialty trainees. She enjoys working as a generalist and has interests in student medicine and women's health.

Prof. Steve Field CBE FRCGP is a GP at the Bellevue Medical Centre in inner-city Birmingham and the immediate past Chairman of Council, Royal College of General Practitioners. Steve is Chairman of the NHS Future Forum, which was launched by the Prime Minister in 2011 and the Deputy National Clinical Director (Health Inequalities) of the National Commissioning Board. He is currently leading a national consultation on the NHS Constitution and chairing the National Inclusion Health Board, which focuses on improving the health outcomes of vulnerable groups, including the homeless. He is Honorary Professor, Medical Education, at the University of Warwick, Honorary Professor in the School of Medicine at the University of Birmingham, and a member of faculty at the Harvard Macy Institute, Harvard University, in Boston, Massachusetts. Steve has published many books and papers on GP education and training, and, in 2010, was awarded the CBE for Services to Medicine.

Foreword to the First Edition

Isn't it strange? If you meet someone socially for the first time and tell them you are a doctor, there is an awful inevitability about what they will say next – 'Are you a specialist or just a GP?' It is that use of the word 'just' that causes the heart to sink – probably in the same way that patients feel their hearts sink when we say their condition is 'just a virus'.

But being a GP is hugely complex. There is something breathtakingly illogical about the way that society generally bestows the highest prestige on those whose area of expertise is smallest, and vice versa. But the undeniable truth is that being a GP is an extraordinarily complex task. After all, patients can, and do, bring us problems of every imaginable dimension, and expect us to have an answer.

The RCGP's magnificent new curriculum for GP training demonstrates the enormity of the task facing family doctors. No one will ever again be able to describe general practice as the simple option, but demonstrating this complexity brings its own problems. Faced with the whole curriculum, many doctors might think they need a simpler career choice – like cardio-thoracic surgery.

And so a book like this is invaluable. This book has two main purposes: it makes the curriculum accessible by condensing it into its core educational material, and it provides practical guidance both on how to learn and how to teach it. Whilst primarily aimed at trainees, parts are of real value to GP educators as well. The authors have deliberately tried to keep the approach pragmatic and point readers towards useful sources of information or practical approaches to learning.

The first half of the book is called 'The Curriculum Guide' and it contains chapters on the background and development of the curriculum, how it is organised, how to learn and teach it, and how to prepare for the new MRCGP assessments. The second part is 'The Condensed Curriculum' and contains the chapters describing and interpreting the first curriculum statement, *Being a General Practitioner*, which explores the core competences of general practice.

General practice needs this book. But, much more importantly and indirectly, so do our patients. After all, high-quality general practice is of vital importance to patients everywhere. GPs really do make a difference.

Prof. David Haslam CBE FRCP FRCGP FFPH
Former President, Royal College of General Practitioners

Foreword to the Second Edition

As GPs, we believe that all patients, families and carers, regardless of background and age, deserve access to high-quality, safe and comprehensive health care.

The idea of caring for the whole person lies at the heart of our vision for the health service. Working within their communities, GPs must learn to assess, plan and deliver services to accommodate local needs, providing both acute and ongoing patient care for an increasing range of problems. All care must be tailored to the individual with careful consideration of co-morbidities and social context; to achieve high-quality care, GPs require a wide array of expert attributes and skills.

The RCGP curriculum captures the broad array of knowledge, skills and expertise that doctors need to care for patients in their homes and communities, working in partnership with other professionals, and ensuring that the care they provide is effective, integrated and holistic.

But given the growing complexity of the GP's role, getting to grips with the curriculum and the MRCGP exams can seem a daunting prospect for many doctors. This book helps both learners and educators achieve this goal by making the curriculum more accessible: condensing it into its core educational material and providing practical tips and advice on how to learn and teach it. As a tool for lifelong learning, this book is also an invaluable guide for tutors, CPD leads, appraisers and GPs preparing for appraisal and revalidation.

With advances in medical management, our ageing population and the increased complexity of primary care, the challenges facing our profession have never been greater; this book will help every new GP develop his or her full role as a generalist and prepare for an exciting and challenging career in the changing NHS.

Prof. Clare Gerada MBE FRCP FRCGP
Chair of Council, Royal College of General Practitioners

Acknowledgements

We would like to thank all the many talented and hard-working colleagues who have contributed to the ongoing development of the RCGP curriculum and MRCGP assessments since their introduction in 2007.

Especially, we would like to acknowledge and highlight the work of the curriculum guardians, the members of the Curriculum Development Committee, the MRCGP Blueprinting and Assessment Groups, and the Postgraduate Training and Professional Development Boards.

We would like to thank the members of the assessment team who kindly contributed their time and expertise to helping us expand and update MRCGP sections within this book, including Amar Rughani, Sue Rendel, Carol Blow, Jane Mamelok and Kamila Hawthorne.

Finally, we would like to thank all of you who supported the first edition of this book – without you this second edition would not have been possible.

What's in this guide?

Part I: The curriculum guide   *Page*

1   Introducing the curriculum   3
What the curriculum is all about, who it is intended for, how
it has been developed, how it is kept up to date and how GP
training is organised, spiral learning, the apprenticeship
model and the role of the trainer.

2   Understanding the curriculum   11
How the curriculum is structured, what's in a curriculum
statement, the core areas of competence and the essential
application features, the relationship between the new core,
contextual and clinical example statements, and also how
the old statements and the new ones map across.

3   Learning and teaching the curriculum   17
How GPs learn, learning from experience, reflective and
self-directed learning, finding out what you need to learn,
problem-based learning in general practice, learning complex
skills, learning in groups, learning from other health professionals, planning activities with the curriculum, learning in
secondary care, giving and receiving feedback, keeping a
learning portfolio.

4   Succeeding at the MRCGP   37
How the MRCGP assessments were developed, the MRCGP
competency areas, how these relate to the curriculum, getting
to grips with the three assessments – the Applied Knowledge
Test (AKT), the Clinical Skills Assessment (CSA) and the
Workplace-Based Assessment (WPBA) – using the ePortfolio, collecting the required evidence, making good reflective
entries, using the assessment tools and completing the interim
and final training reviews.

Part II: The condensed curriculum   *Page*

How we condensed the RCGP curriculum into this book.

5   The core curriculum   **77**
The areas of competence of general practice, how these were identified, a quick overview, the six areas of competence and the three essential application features explained in detail, our tips on how to learn them.

6   The applied knowledge   **131**
How to use the condensed curriculum statements and our tips for learning them; the condensed knowledge, skills, know-how and useful educational resources.

6a. The contextual statements

2.01   *The GP Consultation in Practice*   **136**

2.02   *Patient Safety and Quality of Care*   **143**

2.03   *The GP in the Wider Professional Environment*   **151**

2.04   *Enhancing Professional Knowledge*   **156**

6b. The clinical example statements

3.01   *Healthy People: promoting health and preventing disease*   **165**

3.02   *Genetics in Primary Care*   **172**

3.03   *Care of Acutely Ill People*   **178**

3.04   *Care of Children and Young People*   **187**

3.05   *Care of Older Adults*   **195**

3.06   *Women's Health*   **200**

3.07   *Men's Health*   **208**

3.08   *Sexual Health*   **214**

3.09   *End-of-Life Care*   **223**

3.10   *Care of People with Mental Health Problems*   **228**

Page

3.11	*Care of People with Intellectual Disability*	**235**
3.12	*Cardiovascular Health*	**240**
3.13	*Digestive Health*	**245**
3.14	*Care of People Who Misuse Drugs and Alcohol*	**250**
3.15	*Care of People with ENT, Oral and Facial Problems*	**256**
3.16	*Care of People with Eye Problems*	**262**
3.17	*Care of People with Metabolic Problems*	**267**
3.18	*Care of People with Neurological Problems*	**273**
3.19	*Respiratory Health*	**278**
3.20	*Care of People with Musculoskeletal Problems*	**284**
3.21	*Care of People with Skin Problems*	**292**

Part III: Appendices and index

**Appendix 1: Getting the most from
specialty-based placements**   **303**
Lists the posts and placements commonly undertaken
in GP training programmes and signposts to the most
relevant parts of the curriculum to help guide training.

**Appendix 2: MRCGP Consultation Observation Tool
(COT) criteria**   **315**
Summary of the MRCGP criteria for assessing
videoed consultations.

**Appendix 3: Common GP topics mapped to the
relevant curriculum statements**   **317**
Indexed list that enables you to find where a topic
appears in the curriculum.

Index   **329**

Part I

The curriculum guide

1 Introducing the curriculum

What is the RCGP curriculum?

The Royal College of General Practitioners (RCGP) Curriculum has been developed to guide doctors through their specialty training and career-long development in general practice. It is an educational document designed to help learners develop the wide-ranging knowledge, clinical skills, communication techniques and professional attitudes considered essential for a doctor practising in primary care in the modern UK National Health Service.

Is it meant for me?

The curriculum has been designed for four main groups.

First and foremost, the curriculum is intended to meet the educational needs of *doctors in training for UK general practice*. For the first time ever, it presents an official view of the core knowledge, skills, attitudes and expertise that a doctor needs to learn and develop to become a competent GP. It takes the broad principles of the General Medical Council's *Good Medical Practice* document,[1] and applies them directly to everyday general practice.

Second, the curriculum is a useful guide for *GP educators*. It forms a framework for trainers, course organisers and other GP educators to plan their training and mentoring, and to design their local educational programmes. The curriculum is designed to form a reliable benchmark against which the performance of new GPs can be assessed at the end of their training, and also to inform the design of the assessments that will be used in the revalidation of established GPs.

Third, the curriculum has been developed to support the continuous learning that occurs throughout a *practising GP's* professional lifetime, as the practitioner moves from being a competent GP to becoming an expert. It acts as an educational framework for revalidation, the five-yearly process by which every GP must prove he or she meets the standards required for re-licensing.

Fourth, the curriculum is intended for *academics* and for those interested in educational research and the development of GP training. The curriculum describes an evidence-based view of contemporary general practice and will aid the continuing development of general practice as a generalist medical discipline.

The initial development of the curriculum

The curriculum was developed by the Education Department of the Royal College of General Practitioners (RCGP), with input from a broad range of people and organisations, including representatives from a variety of backgrounds. This included working GPs, trainers, other primary care educators, secondary care experts, GP trainees and members of the public.

A strong evidence-based approach was taken to the development of the curriculum. A literature review was commissioned from the Centre for Research into Medical and Dental Education at the University of Birmingham, which has published widely in this area.[2] At the same time, an extensive consultation exercise was carried out, which included:

- a national questionnaire survey of the views of trainees and GP educators

- meetings with patient representatives, members of the public and GP trainees

- focus groups and presentations at national and international conferences on GP education to share findings and explore ideas.

After this process was complete, the first curriculum statement was written: *Being a General Practitioner*. This formed the template for the rest of the curriculum. Each statement was coordinated by a GP with particular expertise in that particular field. The statements were then circulated in draft form to GPs, educators, patient representatives, members of the public, trainees and specialist interest groups within the RCGP. They were also posted on the RCGP website. There was a period of formal consultation and revision before finally the whole bundle of statements was approved by the Postgraduate Medical Education and Training Board (PMETB), the relevant regulatory body at the time, whose functions have since been taken over by the General Medical Council (GMC).

Keeping the curriculum up to date

General practice is a constantly changing profession and the curriculum must be adaptable to the ever-changing circumstances in primary care, such as changes that come about as a result of new government policy or unexpected national events.

The curriculum is reviewed continuously, by a process that involves annual reviews of feedback submitted by a wide range of users and special interest groups, reviews of assessment data from the MRCGP examinations, and commissioned research. Each statement in the curriculum has a named clinician, known as a 'guardian', who has responsibility for that statement. Guardians are responsible for the monitoring of their statement and for proposing any changes.

GP training in the UK is organised by local regions, known as deaneries. Each deanery collects a range of data every year to feed into the curriculum review process, including quality assurance reports, GP trainee performance data, national exit survey data and the views of local educators in the deanery.

GP educators, trainees, members of the public and patients are closely involved in the ongoing monitoring of the curriculum. All specialty trainees complete an exit survey on the completion of their training, and trainees, educators and patient representatives are involved in the group that approves changes to the curriculum.

The 2012 curriculum revision

Based on feedback gathered from users since its launch in 2007, the structure and presentation of curriculum was revised in 2012. The language used in the documents was also modified, in order to make them more user-friendly.

We will describe the new structure of the curriculum in the next chapter, 'Understanding the curriculum'.

The role of the curriculum in GP training

The curriculum describes the core competences that a doctor is expected to master by the end of his or her specialty training programme for general practice. This means that the days are gone when a new GP trainee spends weeks searching fruitlessly for an official opinion on 'what a GP needs to know'. GPs in training can now focus their efforts instead on developing the identified core knowledge, attitudes and skills of general practice. It also enables trainees working in hospital-based training posts to identify which areas of their work will be most relevant to their subsequent role in primary care.

How the curriculum is applied to individual learners will vary considerably from person to person, and it is extremely important for GPs in training to develop their adult learning skills and to identify their individual learning needs.

As well as being particularly useful for current trainees and their educational supervisors, the curriculum is relevant to a much wider group of people. The curriculum has a role to play for every GP who is actively wishing to maintain good standards of professional practice – providing a blueprint for Continuing Professional Development (CPD) and lifelong medical education.

How GP training is organised

The GP Specialty Training Programme, which is covered by the curriculum, currently runs for *three years* from the end of the two-year Foundation Programme to the award of the Certificate of Completion of Training, when a doctor qualifies as a GP. During this time, GPs in training are officially referred to as 'GP specialty trainees'. If they are also members of the RCGP (which all but a handful are), then they are also known as 'Associates-in-Training'.

Places on GP training programmes are awarded through a national selection scheme. Each training programme has a Programme Director, who has responsibility for the sequence of posts that make up the programme and the quality of the training that is provided. Educators based in primary care and secondary care help directors to deliver the training. The emphasis is on learning in the workplace, although some teaching is arranged more formally with courses and day-release programmes, including a number of mandatory courses (e.g. child safeguarding). Ongoing mentoring and educational supervision takes place throughout the training programme.

Figure 1.1

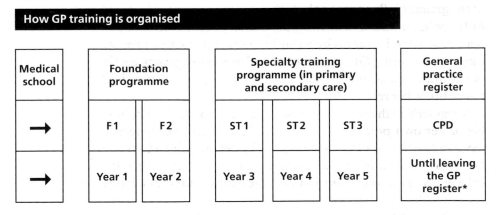

How GP training is organised

Medical school	Foundation programme		Specialty training programme (in primary and secondary care)			General practice register
	F1	F2	ST1	ST2	ST3	CPD
	Year 1	Year 2	Year 3	Year 4	Year 5	Until leaving the GP register*

F = foundation   ST = specialty training   CPD = Continuing Professional Development
*usually at retirement age, unless you are lucky enough to win the lottery!

Work is currently underway to develop a new four-year GP specialty training programme with increased focus on child health, mental health, coordination of care and leadership.[3] However, at the time of writing, a start date for this enhanced and extended GP training programme had not yet been finalised.

Apprenticeship and the role of the GP trainer

The primary relationship in GP training exists between the trainee (the learner) and his or her educational supervisor (the trainer). It is at the heart of the teaching and learning process, whereby trainees acquire and develop the knowledge, skills and attitudes needed to become an effective GP. The relationship is embedded in daily professional working practice: an apprenticeship that blends daily professional work with education to enable the development of expertise.[4,i] It is not uncommon for this relationship to continue after formal training has ended.

The GP trainer forms the bedrock of general practice training in the UK. The role is complex, challenging and diverse; it encompasses the responsibilities of critical friend, supervisor, educator, assessor, mentor, pastoral carer and role model. These roles are complex and may, at times, come into conflict. It is the primary responsibility of the educational supervisor to oversee and support the specialty trainee's educational progress throughout their training programme. To do this, a trainer must have the appropriate professional attributes, personal qualities and training required for the task.

A specialty trainee will derive most of his or her useful learning from seeing and contributing to good-quality patient care. One of the greatest influences on the trainees is the example presented by his or her trainer as a doctor – the trainee's role model. For this reason, a GP trainer must be an enthusiastic, competent, communicative and caring GP, working in a well-organised practice.[ii] He or she must also be expected to know and accept the responsibilities of his or her role.

A trainer's enthusiasm for general practice must also apply to his or her own personal learning and his or her willingness to develop further as a clinical teacher. Trainers require additional knowledge and skills over and above those of their non-teaching colleagues. Trainers' contribution to learning activities outside

---

i Lave and Wenger define apprenticeship as the development of professional expertise through 'legitimate peripheral participation in a community of practice'. See Lave J, Wenger E. *Situated Learning: legitimate peripheral participation.* Cambridge: Cambridge University Press, 1991.

ii The ability to leap over tall buildings is optional!

the practice is often a good illustration of a wider commitment to education. Trainers must devote time to prepare carefully for their training responsibilities and may benefit from wider teaching experience, for example with medical students or other health professionals. They should be willing to be appraised by their peers as this encourages their trainees to adopt a similar critical approach to their work.

Spiral learning and the curriculum

Spiral learning involves revisiting the same areas of the curriculum on several occasions over time.[5] This may mean reviewing individual statements, competences or even individual learning outcomes more than once, each time focusing in greater depth and complexity. This is similar to an aircraft descending in a spiral as it prepares to land – the concept will be familiar to anyone who has been in a plane descending over London. As the plane repeatedly circles round, lower and lower each time, the familiar landmarks and buildings can be seen in increasing detail.

Each time an area of the curriculum is revisited, learners:

- review what was previously learned

- reinforce the recognition of important patterns (e.g. patterns of health and disease)

- gain a greater awareness of what determines their decisions

- expand their range of management options

- achieve a more complex understanding (e.g. enabling them to tailor their responses to the individual patient and to offer greater choice).

The informal curriculum

While the RCGP has invested considerable energy into developing an official curriculum for GP training, the 'informal curriculum' is also an important component of a trainee's learning. The informal curriculum is the term used to describe what trainees learn from a variety of sources and interactions while taking part in extracurricular activities.[6] The trainer has a role in ensuring that there is sufficient flexibility and time for the specialty registrar to make the most of educational opportunities available outside of work and the formal teaching programme.

The hidden curriculum

The 'hidden curriculum' describes what the trainee learns but the trainer did not set out to teach! The degree of professionalism exhibited by role models can exert an important influence on a learner's professional development over time. Doctors should be aware that this will have already occurred from previous experiences – trainers may encounter a trainee who encountered poor role models during his or her education or early medical training. Many doctors have had personal experience of teachers who intimidate and humiliate their students, which discourages participation and has a negative effect on learning.

All doctors should be aware that the way their colleagues are treated may influence the way they, in turn, will learn to behave. A doctor may not consider this when making a demeaning remark about a patient, a patient's relative, a nurse or a colleague, even if it is not meant seriously. We need to create an environment where the 'hidden curriculum' reinforces, rather than undermines, our professional ideals.

How to use the curriculum in everyday general practice

This is why we have written this guide.

At first glance, the biggest difficulty with using the curriculum is its size and extremely broad coverage. The full curriculum contains many hundreds of learning outcomes! However, once you start to examine the curriculum more closely, you will discover it is not quite as overwhelming as it may at first seem.

You will have noticed that this guide is a fraction of the size of the full curriculum. So how it is possible to compress such a large, comprehensive document into a condensed guide? This is explained in the following chapter, which describes how the curriculum itself is organised and what the fancy educational words like 'competence' and 'learning outcome' mean in everyday general practice.

References

1   General Medical Council. *Good Medical Practice*. London: GMC, 2012, www.gmc-uk.org.

2   Bullock A, Burke S, Wall D. Curriculum and assessment in higher specialist training. *Medical Teacher* 2004; **26(2)**: 174–7.

3 Gerada C, Riley B, Simon C. *Preparing the Future GP: the case for enhanced GP training*. London: RCGP, 2012, www.rcgp.org.uk/policy/rcgp-policy-areas/enhanced-and-extended-speciality-training-in-general-practice.aspx/ [accessed May 2012].

4 Lave J, Wenger E. *Situated Learning: legitimate peripheral participation*. Cambridge: Cambridge University Press, 1991.

5 Harden R, Stamper N: What is a spiral curriculum? *Medical Teacher* 1999; **21(2)**: 141–3.

6 Mohanna K, Wall D, Chambers R. *Teaching Made Easy*. Oxford: Radcliffe Medical Press, 2003.

2 Understanding the curriculum

The curriculum framework

In order to understand how the curriculum works, and how to use it for learning and teaching, you need to understand how it is constructed. This involves familiarising yourself with the curriculum framework (i.e. its basic anatomy).

Figure 2.1

The anatomy of the RCGP curriculum

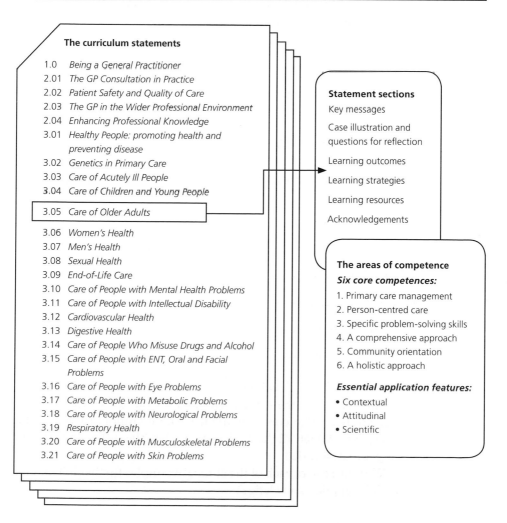

The curriculum statements

1.0 *Being a General Practitioner*
2.01 *The GP Consultation in Practice*
2.02 *Patient Safety and Quality of Care*
2.03 *The GP in the Wider Professional Environment*
2.04 *Enhancing Professional Knowledge*
3.01 *Healthy People: promoting health and preventing disease*
3.02 *Genetics in Primary Care*
3.03 *Care of Acutely Ill People*
3.04 *Care of Children and Young People*
3.05 *Care of Older Adults*
3.06 *Women's Health*
3.07 *Men's Health*
3.08 *Sexual Health*
3.09 *End-of-Life Care*
3.10 *Care of People with Mental Health Problems*
3.11 *Care of People with Intellectual Disability*
3.12 *Cardiovascular Health*
3.13 *Digestive Health*
3.14 *Care of People Who Misuse Drugs and Alcohol*
3.15 *Care of People with ENT, Oral and Facial Problems*
3.16 *Care of People with Eye Problems*
3.17 *Care of People with Metabolic Problems*
3.18 *Care of People with Neurological Problems*
3.19 *Respiratory Health*
3.20 *Care of People with Musculoskeletal Problems*
3.21 *Care of People with Skin Problems*

Statement sections
Key messages
Case illustration and questions for reflection
Learning outcomes
Learning strategies
Learning resources
Acknowledgements

The areas of competence
Six core competences:
1. Primary care management
2. Person-centred care
3. Specific problem-solving skills
4. A comprehensive approach
5. Community orientation
6. A holistic approach

Essential application features:
• Contextual
• Attitudinal
• Scientific

The core statement: Being a General Practitioner

The core of the curriculum is explained in the statement *Being a General Practitioner*. This contains a description of the knowledge, skills, attitudes and behaviours required of a modern GP. This statement is the heart of the curriculum and we will explore it in more detail in Chapter 5, 'The core curriculum'.

The contextual statements

The four 'contextual statements' (statements 2.01 to 2.04) consider certain aspects of general practice in greater depth. They focus mainly on the professional skills required for everyday general practice, such as consultation skills, patient safety skills, adult learning skills and evidence-based practice. We will explore these statements further in Chapter 6, 'The applied knowledge'.

The clinical examples

The 21 'clinical examples' (statements 3.01 to 3.21) apply the general skills in the core curriculum to a range of clinical topics, such as *Cardiovascular Health*. Some of the clinical examples focus on population groups, as in the statements on *Care of Children and Young People* and *Men's Health*.

Each of the clinical example statements follows the same basic template:

- key messages
- case illustration and questions for reflection
- learning outcomes
- learning strategies
- learning resources
- acknowledgements.

To use an analogy, each clinical example is like a different breed of dog: each has the same basic features but a slightly different appearance. The core statement is the common ancestor (the wolf) from which all the clinical examples (the different breeds of dog) are descended.

We will explore each of the clinical examples further in Chapter 6, 'The applied knowledge'.

Accessing the curriculum

The full curriculum statements can be freely accessed on the RCGP website (www.rcgp.org.uk/curriculum) and are also available in the RCGP Trainee ePortfolio (https://eportfolio.rcgp.org.uk). You may find it useful to refer to the curriculum statements while reading this chapter.

Some of the statements describe the professional and managerial aspects of general practice, some describe the care of special groups of people and some describe specific clinical topics.

Table 2.1

The RCGP curriculum statements [1]		
Core statement	1.0	*Being a General Practitioner*
Contextual statements	2.01	*The GP Consultation in Practice*
	2.02	*Patient Safety and Quality of Care*
	2.03	*The GP in the Wider Professional Environment*
	2.04	*Enhancing Professional Knowledge*
Clinical examples	3.01	*Healthy People: promoting health and preventing disease*
	3.02	*Genetics in Primary Care*
	3.03	*Care of Acutely Ill People*
	3.04	*Care of Children and Young People*
	3.05	*Care of Older Adults*
	3.06	*Women's Health*
	3.07	*Men's Health*
	3.08	*Sexual Health*
	3.09	*End-of-Life Care*
	3.10	*Care of People with Mental Health Problems*
	3.11	*Care of People with Intellectual Disability*
	3.12	*Cardiovascular Health*
	3.13	*Digestive Health*
	3.14	*Care of People Who Misuse Drugs and Alcohol*

Continued over

3.15 *Care of People with ENT, Oral and Facial Problems*

3.16 *Care of People with Eye Problems*

3.17 *Care of People with Metabolic Problems*

3.18 *Care of People with Neurological Problems*

3.19 *Respiratory Health*

3.20 *Care of People with Musculoskeletal Problems*

3.21 *Care of People with Skin Problems*

The learning outcomes

The key part of each curriculum statement is the learning outcomes section. Each individual *learning outcome* is a brief description of a specific item of knowledge, skill, attitude or expertise that a GP must develop, in order to be competent. In some of the curriculum statements, these individual learning outcomes have been organised into groups, which together make up an everyday GP task. The ability to do an everyday task is known as a *competency*.[i]

Table 2.2

An example of a competency and its associated learning outcomes

Competency	1.1	To manage primary contact with patients and deal with unselected problems
Learning outcomes		*This requires you to:*
	•	understand the epidemiology of problems presenting in primary care
	•	master an approach that allows easy access for patients with unselected problems
	•	use an organised approach to the management of chronic conditions
	•	know the conditions encountered in primary care and their treatment

i There are many academic definitions of *competency/competencies/competences* and debating these can entertain educationalists for many hours. In this book, we will try to keep things simple!

To *achieve* competence, a doctor must first master the individual learning outcomes and develop the ability to put these together purposefully. This is in order to perform the task to a professional standard.

Table 2.3

The curriculum phrase book	
Area of competence	One of the six areas of competence of general practice: primary care management, person-centred care, specific problem-solving skills, a comprehensive approach, community orientation and a holistic approach. See Chapter 5, 'The core curriculum', for more details
Competency	An everyday task that a GP must be able to perform to a professional standard (usually requiring mastery of a group of several learning outcomes)
Curriculum statement	One of the documents that together make up the RCGP Curriculum for Specialty Training for General Practice
Essential application feature	A fundamental aspect of general practice that applies to an individual GP and determines how he or she applies acquired knowledge and skills to a real-life situation: contextual, scientific and attitudinal. See Chapter 5, 'The core curriculum', for more details
Learning outcome	A specific piece of knowledge, skill, attitude or area of expertise that a GP should acquire

The knowledge base

One of the most appealing aspects of general practice is its enormous variety and breadth, and it will never be possible to write a list of every condition you might need to learn over the course of your career – the ability to seek out and appraise new knowledge when required is a fundamental skill in general practice. On this basis, the RCGP curriculum is intended as a foundation to a career in general practice and not an exhaustive list of topics.

The curriculum learning outcomes include various kinds of knowledge-based information, such as:

- symptoms
- common and important conditions
- investigations

- treatment

- emergency care

- prevention.

To assist your learning, we (the authors of this book) have presented a knowledge base for general practice within this guide, drawn from the content in the curriculum and our own clinical experience. This is located in Chapter 6, 'The applied knowledge'.

References

1   Royal College of General Practitioners revised curriculum statements, 2012, www.rcgp-curriculum.org.uk/rcgp_curriculum_documents.aspx [accessed May 2012].

3 Learning and teaching the curriculum

How GPs learn

There are a number of key principles that make learning more effective for adults, which have been identified from many years of research. These principles of adult learning are particularly relevant for GPs – if they are applied successfully in general practice, learning will be more successful:

1 GPs learn from experience

Learning in most adults is generally more effective when it is based on real experience rather than abstract theory alone. For a GP, learning from experience involves reflecting on (i.e. 'thinking about') events that occur in daily practice, considering why these feel significant, addressing any learning needs that arise and formulating a new approach that can be adopted in the future. Then, the next time a similar situation recurs, the GP's response will be different; this leads to another new experience, a further opportunity for reflection, and so on. This reflective learning cycle can repeat *ad infinitum* and each time it occurs something new can be learnt. This is the cycle of experiential and reflective learning.[1]

2 GPs like to direct their own learning

Most adults like to feel in charge of their lives and the same applies to their learning, although there are times when we want to be told what learning activities to do rather than find out for ourselves. This is particularly the case when a learner is under stress or adjusting to a new learning environment. Specialty trainees (GP) who are just starting out in general practice often initially request a considerable amount of direction from their trainers and course organisers, although they tend to take more and more control of their learning as their experience and confidence grows. This principle is referred to as self-directed learning.[2]

3 GPs learn what they need to learn

For many GPs, their readiness to learn is often strongly related to how relevant they perceive a learning activity to be to the tasks they perform in their day-to-day role. In other words, learning based on the curriculum needs to feel relevant to learning how to be a GP, passing the MRCGP assessments, or getting through appraisal and revalidation – or many learners will lose interest. This principle is known as needs-based learning.

4 GPs learn how to solve problems

Traditionally, lessons at school are categorised into subjects. In medical school, we call these 'topics' or 'specialties'. Unfortunately for GPs, however, patients in the real world do not often present with their complaints neatly categorised. A competent GP must learn to apply his or her medical expertise effectively to daily situations, based on the underlying theoretical medical knowledge and theory he or she has previously acquired. This is the principle behind problem-based learning.[3]

Learning from experience in general practice

The learning acquired in medical school that is based on theoretical topics is an essential foundation for general practice, but this form of education is traditionally focused on learning *about medicine* rather than learning *how to be a doctor*. This is similar to the difference between learning the mechanics of how a car works and learning how to drive. One of the best ways to learn to be a competent GP is by undertaking learning activities based in real-life, supervised situations, and by addressing the unpredictable problems that arise when seeing patients. This is the rationale for developing training programmes based on problem-based learning (also referred to as problem-centred learning).

Consultation analysis

The development of good consulting skills is a key objective of GP training and it is therefore crucial that every trainee's consultations are observed and analysed on a regular basis (see statement 2.01 *The GP Consultation in Practice*). This can be done by direct observation by the trainer sitting in with the trainee or by videoing the surgery and watching it back later.

Video consultations formed a major component of the old summative assessment system and, through the new MRCGP consultation observation tool (COT),[i] it remains an important part of

---

i See Chapter 4, 'Succeeding at the MRCGP', for more information on COT and other assessment tools.

teaching the curriculum. Videoing of consultations should begin as soon as possible after GP training has commenced, as it is a superb method of identifying learning needs and improving communication skills.

Regular opportunities for specialty trainees to sit in and observe their trainer and other experienced GPs are part of a well-rounded training experience. Holding joint surgeries with a variety of practitioners enables trainees to:

- gain real-time feedback on their consultation performance

- see new techniques and approaches being used

- take advantage of opportunities for case-based discussion

- arrange to review any patients causing them particular difficulty or concern with an experienced colleague.

Undertaking joint surgeries, preferably with a number of different clinicians, provides variety and exposes the trainee to a range of alternative consulting styles and techniques.[4]

Doctors often gain their first experience of consulting in general practice while sitting in with their trainer and observing other, established GPs and primary care professionals. These early experiences may be very influential in determining the behaviours that a fledgling GP will adopt in his or her own professional practice. As time progresses, these supervised surgeries are gradually replaced by unsupervised surgeries, initially supported with formal 'debriefing' time.

Reflective learning

Reflection is an important stage of the learning process in general practice. This requires learners to successfully develop the skills of reflection *on practice* and reflection *in practice*.[5,6] Reflection *on practice* involves thinking back to a situation in the past, such as a consultation, and recalling what happened and considering the feelings generated at that time by the experience. Both the events and the feelings are analysed and explored to identify any significant learning points (Description → Feelings → Analysis → Conclusion). The purpose of analysing the experience in this way is to transform it from a vague emotional memory into usable knowledge and helpful understanding that can be adopted in future practice.

Figure 3.1

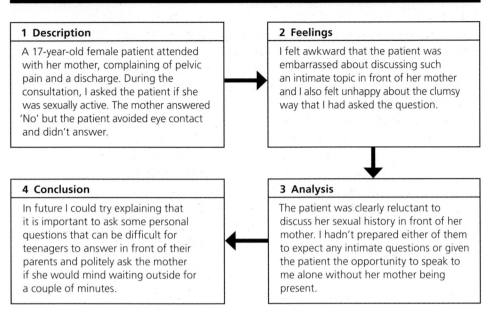

An example of reflection on practice

1 Description

A 17-year-old female patient attended with her mother, complaining of pelvic pain and a discharge. During the consultation, I asked the patient if she was sexually active. The mother answered 'No' but the patient avoided eye contact and didn't answer.

2 Feelings

I felt awkward that the patient was embarrassed about discussing such an intimate topic in front of her mother and I also felt unhappy about the clumsy way that I had asked the question.

4 Conclusion

In future I could try explaining that it is important to ask some personal questions that can be difficult for teenagers to answer in front of their parents and politely ask the mother if she would mind waiting outside for a couple of minutes.

3 Analysis

The patient was clearly reluctant to discuss her sexual history in front of her mother. I hadn't prepared either of them to expect any intimate questions or given the patient the opportunity to speak to me alone without her mother being present.

Reflection *in practice* involves reflecting in real time, while a situation is ongoing, and adjusting your behaviour accordingly. For example, a GP with underdeveloped reflective skills may experience feelings of anger during a challenging consultation and respond by growing increasingly angry him or herself, only to regret this behaviour afterwards. A GP with highly developed reflective skills would recognise these growing feelings of anger and take action to deal with them appropriately, possibly by sharing his or her feelings with the patient: 'I would like to help you but I'm finding it difficult to think of how to do this as I am feeling increasingly frustrated myself. . . .'

GPs with strong reflective preferences may spend a lot of time ruminating on past events, whereas those with activist tendencies may find reflection more of an uphill struggle. In either case, it is important that reflection should be a constructive process with tangible rather than imaginary benefits. Reflection can be aided by a variety of techniques. Natural introverts and reflectors may prefer personal reflective diaries and one-to-one debriefing sessions. Those with more extrovert and activist preferences, however, may prefer to reflect through discussion with their peers, debates in learning groups and direct feedback.[7]

Self-awareness assessments

There are a number of techniques available to aid learners gain a deeper understanding of their personality, educational preferences and approaches to learning. Most have been developed by educational or organisational psychologists and are questionnaire-based tools, usually available on a commercial basis. They include those concentrating on personality styles, e.g. Myers–Briggs,[8] and learning styles, e.g. Honey and Mumford.[9]

The *Honey and Mumford's Learning Styles Questionnaire*[9] can be a useful tool to help a learner understand his or her learning style preferences in terms of four broad categories – *Activists, Theorists, Pragmatists* and *Reflectors*. Many trainers encourage their trainees to undertake the assessment as part of the induction programme. The questionnaire is available online and takes about 10–20 minutes. At the end of the session the learner receives a report of his or her current learning style preferences as well as information about the types of learning activities in keeping with these.

Most people display a mixture of all four styles, although one or two tend to be dominant. Educators tend to replicate their learning style preferences in the teaching styles they adopt. Sometimes a trainer and trainee will happen to share the same learning preferences; this can result in a harmonious educational partnership, although it risks a degree of over-comfort and possible collusion, which can potentially inhibit the development of the less preferred learning styles in the trainee. More visible educational difficulties can arise when there is a large mismatch in preferences between learner and teacher – for example, a strongly reflective trainer and an activist trainee can have quite different opinions on the best ways to learn!

Self-directed learning in general practice

An effective self-directed approach to learning involves far more than spending an hour each week in a tutorial discussing any interesting patients that spring to mind! A self-directed approach actually requires a lot of planning and organisation; tutorials and other educational activities should be planned in advance to create a personalised programme of educational experiences. In other words, each learning activity should be designed to meet specific objectives based on the learner's identified learning needs, and the particular educational activities chosen should be tailored to complement the learner's individual learning preferences.

It is unrealistic, however, to expect new specialty trainees to arrive in general practice with all the learning skills required to adopt a fully self-directed approach to their learning. Most experienced trainers recognise this and arrange an induction programme involving a number of prearranged educational activities for the first few weeks, encouraging their trainees to take on more responsibility for managing their own learning as their self-directed learning skills develop.

The ability to create a Personal Development Plan (PDP) is an important aspect of self-directed professional learning and this key skill is increasingly important for GPs undergoing annual appraisal and revalidation. More tips and advice on this are included below.

Learning what you need to learn

One of the first questions every new GP trainee asks is 'What do I need to learn to be a GP?' Although many answers to this question exist, very few of these are particularly helpful to the learner.

- 'Learn a bit about everything ...'
- 'Only you can decide what you need to learn ...'
- 'Learn the RCGP curriculum ...'

General practice is a very broad specialty and the curriculum is similarly broad – the first step every GP in training must do when planning learning is to identify his or her learning needs in order to set some priorities.

It is important for the educational supervisor and trainee to meet regularly to organise a plan to identify and address learning needs. It is useful to begin with a review of the past experience and the knowledge and skills that the trainee has so far acquired. There are many aids for the trainer to use at the beginning of training to help identify learning needs and many of these can be used at intervals throughout the training programme.

Learners can themselves identify their individual learning needs through a large number of educational activities. Some of these are listed in Table 3.1.

Table 3.1

Popular activities for identifying learning needs in general practice

1 Activities performed by the learner
- Reflective practice
- Keeping a reflective diary of consultations
- Keeping a log of referrals and investigations
- Reflection on learning experiences
- Reflection on an issue at intervals over time
- Self-assessment of knowledge and skills
- Completing a confidence rating scale
- Reviewing the outcomes of referrals
- Reviewing a targeted or random selection of case notes
- Self-directed learning activities
- Reading journal articles and textbooks
- Completing e-learning modules
- Viewing the world wide web/TV/media

2 Activities performed with others
- Learning needs identified with patients
- Recording difficulties arising in day-to-day practice
- Asking for informal feedback from patients
- Getting patients to complete satisfaction questionnaires
- Video analysis of consultations
- Learning needs identified by educational activities
- Recording learning needs arising out of tutorials
- Identifying learning needs in joint surgeries
- Learning needs identified by problem-based learning
- Formative assessment and feedback
- Learning needs identified with peers
- Creating presentations for peers
- Organising and leading group teaching activities
- Attending courses and educational meetings
- Learning needs identified with the practice team
- Discussing issues arising in practice meetings
- Obtaining 360° feedback from the practice team
- Undertaking a Significant Event Analysis

3 Activities that use the RCGP curriculum
- Learner self-assessment
- Assessing your own competences against the core competences
- Testing your own knowledge against the knowledge base
- Judging your own behaviour against the curriculum outcomes
- Formative assessment based on curriculum competences
- Undertaking Workplace-Based Assessment (WPBA)

Chapters 5 and 6 of this guide, 'The core curriculum' and 'The applied knowledge', have been designed for use as a confidence rating scale. Learners can use them to score themselves on their 'level of confidence' for a comprehensive list of topics drawn from the curriculum. Other examples of confidence rating scales include the Wolverhampton Grid and Manchester Rating Scale.[10] This approach can be useful for a new specialty trainee to start prioritising his or her learning needs, although it is important to remember that a confidence score may not always accurately reflect a true level of ability! Another useful tool for prioritising learning needs are RCGP Scotland's Personal Education Planning (PEP) tools (www.elearning.rcgp.org.uk) – online interactive tests of general practice that identify and map your areas of strength and weakness across the curriculum topics.

Contact with patients will generate many learning needs on a daily basis, particularly at the start of training, which can be recorded in a patient log or learning portfolio. More complex learning needs can be identified by case analysis, consultation analysis (video surgeries) and joint surgeries.

Learning needs identified by patient contact

As doctors have contact with the patients they see each day, they generate many identifiable learning needs. It's important to capture the moment by recording these in a log or in your ePortfolio.

PUNs & DENs is a straightforward system to aid reflective experiential learning, developed in Taunton by Dr Richard Eve.[11] After each consultation, doctors are encouraged to record any patient needs that they felt they had not managed well (PUNs – Patient's Unmet Needs); some of these PUNS are the direct result of the doctor's lack of knowledge or skill (DENs – Doctor's Educational Needs). The trainer can use this method to help the trainee reflect on why the patient's needs went unmet and develop an action plan to address the identified learning needs.

Case analysis is an essential weapon in the learner's armoury. It is a useful tool during a trainee's induction period to identify initial learning needs and may form the basis of many tutorials throughout the three-year training programme. There are a number of types of case analysis:

- problem case analysis – this involves the selection by the trainer or trainee of cases that are interesting, challenging or problematic. Analysing the cases provides an opportunity to discuss the learning needs that arose and how to deal with them

- random case analysis – this is potentially less comfortable and involves randomly selecting cases from surgeries; this enables the trainer to ascertain how the specialty trainee is managing his or her cases and ensure that an appropriate mix of cases is being experienced

- analysis of prescriptions, referrals and critical events – these methods provide a wealth of information on the current knowledge and patient management skills of the developing GP.

Problem-based learning in primary care

Many of the learning needs that arise in daily practice are relatively simple (e.g. a need to find out a simple piece of factual knowledge) and can be simply recorded in a logbook or spreadsheet and dealt with on a daily basis.

With the advent of rapid internet access, a number of web-based resources now exist that can enable GPs to address simple learning needs during the consultation, meaning that learning occurs immediately and feels highly relevant.

Table 3.2

An example of a simple learning need arising during a consultation	
Problem	An 18-year-old student attends with abdominal bloating and intermittent loose stools
Comments	History suggests irritable bowel syndrome, but I decide I ought to exclude coeliac disease – only I can't remember the best blood investigation for this …
Learning need	Learn the best blood test for excluding coeliac disease
Action taken	Looked up on www.gpnotebook.co.uk during the consultation. Best screening test is anti-endomysial antibody test, which has a sensitivity of over 95% in the presence of normal IgA
Outcome	Blood test taken – antibody result is negative with normal IgA, effectively ruling out coeliac disease in this context. Patient is started on anti-spasmodic treatment for irritable bowel syndrome; symptoms much better at review two weeks later!

Problem-based case analysis

Complex cases can form the basis of problem-based discussions in tutorials and group learning. Cases can be selected by random (incorporating the element of surprise) or from a logbook recording the most challenging cases encountered.

Tutorials

Tutorials based on particular topics (e.g. gut problems) have a role when a specific learning need in this area has been identified, and are often most effective when both the trainee and the trainer have had the opportunity to prepare in advance. Once the theoretical knowledge has been covered, it is often very useful to discuss how the knowledge can be applied to real-life cases, as the application of knowledge requires a higher level of learning and it is at this stage when the difficulties often emerge.

Learning complex skills

Learning needs arising from problem-based cases that involve the development of complex GP skills, attitudes or expertise require a more sophisticated approach. This includes communication skills, consultation techniques and dealing with ethical dilemmas.

It is often useful to translate these more complex learning needs into personal learning outcomes. A learning outcome is a brief description of a behaviour or activity that the learner is able to demonstrate, the context where it will be demonstrated, the standard to which it will be performed, and the time scale in which it will be achieved.

Table 3.3

An example of a personal learning outcome	
The activity	I will be able to negotiate shared management plans with patients …
The context	in my everyday consultations …
The standard	to the standard required to practise independently as a GP …
The time scale	by the completion of my GP training

As with curriculum learning outcomes, personal learning outcomes can be further broken down into their component parts – knowledge, attitudes and skills – and these component parts can be addressed as part of a personal learning plan (PLP) involving a range of different learning activities.

Learning in groups

The half-day release courses run by GP training programmes are generally very popular among specialty trainees.[ii] This is partly because learning groups provide important functions that extend far beyond the simple educational aims of the particular group activity. For example, many specialty trainees particularly value the opportunity to meet with fellow trainees in order to share experiences with patients ('horror stories') and chat about how they are tackling their learning. Being a specialty trainee can feel quite isolated at times, especially as few practices are able to take more than one new learner at a time; a weekly meeting with a group of peers performs an important 'housekeeping' function for many trainees (as per Neighbour's five-checkpoint consultation model).[12]

In order to deliver GP education in line with national requirements, training programme directors are offering specialty trainees more say in the planning of their group learning programmes. This is also important to ensure that learning in groups is self-directed and needs based, otherwise the educational activities of the group may become increasingly irrelevant to individual learners.

Research suggests that learning groups are most productive if they are facilitated effectively, although many groups can eventually become productive by themselves if given sufficient time to develop.[13] Many specialty trainees, trainers and newly qualified GPs form their own informal learning groups to help them prepare for assessments or to facilitate continuing professional development.

Group learning can be particularly useful for the shaping of attitudes and also act as professional 'barometers' against which individual GPs may judge their own professional opinions and values. Groups are the perfect setting to debate wider ethical and professional issues, often arising from difficult cases, the learning of which requires the consideration of points of view that are necessarily different from one's own.

---

ii Well anything's better than real work, right?!

Learning from other health professionals

An essential part of being a doctor involves teaching and learning from other health professionals. This is increasingly the case in general practice. A GP may be involved, either directly or indirectly, in educational activities with medical students, Foundation-year doctors, specialty trainees, established GPs and other healthcare professionals and staff members in the practice.

Spending time with other primary healthcare team workers and other related professionals (such as community pharmacists and physios) is often very useful.

Table 3.4

Learning from other healthcare professionals	
Spend time with	**Particularly good for learning**
Practice nurses	Chronic disease management, routine vaccinations and travel immunisations, dressings and wound care, issues that arise when implementing practice protocols or national guidelines, minor illness
District nurses	How to manage chronic disease in the community, dressings and wound care, ulcers, catheterisation and incontinence, local community services, palliative care
Health visitors	Management of common childhood problems such as behavioural difficulties, feeding and toileting, supporting new parents, child protection, vulnerable adults
Community pharmacists	Common prescribing problems, how medications are dispensed, dosette boxes, compliance and concordance
Physiotherapists	How to manage common musculoskeletal complaints, triaging back problems, self-management of back pain

Learning in secondary care

Many acute medical and surgical jobs provide great experience of managing seriously ill patients in hospital. In the UK, however, a GP does not usually spend very long managing a patient who is obviously seriously ill, beyond administering immediate emergency care until an ambulance arrives, or caring for a terminally ill patient at home. A hospital post, therefore, can be a great opportunity for learning how to examine, investigate and manage patients with serious illnesses and for practising specific psycho-motor skills (like joint injections or taking a cervical sample for screening).

Table 3.5

Useful learning opportunities in secondary care	
Spend time in	**Particularly good for learning**
Outpatient clinics	Secondary care management, consulting with patients, how specialists manage specialised conditions, familiarity with serious illness, developing specific clinical and psychomotor skills
Consultant ward-rounds	Bedside teaching and getting consultant feedback on clinical and decision-making skills
Multidisciplinary team meetings	How multidisciplinary teams work together and communicate
Educational meetings	A range of specialist educational topics

GPs must learn how to distinguish patients who *may be seriously ill* and need to go to hospital from the far larger group of patients presenting in the community with symptoms but without serious illness, the vast majority of whom never trouble secondary care. Most jobs in secondary care, therefore, offer relatively poor opportunities for GPs to learn how to examine, investigate and manage symptomatic patients who do not have serious illnesses, and these skills are best honed during the time spent in general practice.

Appendix 1 highlights the learning opportunities which may be available in the common specialty-based placements that make up the early part of many GP specialty training programmes.

Using the curriculum as a teaching resource

The curriculum statements themselves can be used as learning materials to resource a range of educational activities. In addition to the learning outcomes, the individual statements include case scenarios and a considerable amount of background information, and point to some useful sources of further information. As such, curriculum statements form a useful basis for a comprehensive tutorial on a topic.

Box 3.1

Leading a teaching session based on a curriculum statement: a ten-point teaching plan

- Start the session and establish rapport with the learner(s).
- Identify the learners' agenda and the teacher's agenda.
- Review the case scenario at the start of the statement.
- Clarify the main issues and set them in the context of everyday practice.
- Explore the learners' suggestions, challenge preconceptions and give feedback.
- Clarify and record any learning needs that arise.
- Review the outcomes described for each of the areas of competence in the *learning outcomes* section of the statement.
- Identify any unmet learning outcomes.
- Plan future learning activities.
- Summarise and conclude the session.

A list of common primary care topics and their corresponding curriculum statements is included in Appendix 3 of this book.

Using the curriculum to address training difficulties

The curriculum is a competency-based document and has been designed to support the training needs of all GPs. It is a useful tool in addressing common problems that trainees and practising GPs may run into. At one extreme, this might involve assisting a trainer in supporting a trainee who is generally underperforming and, at the other extreme, using the curriculum to stretch the abilities of a high achiever.

Feedback and formative assessment

Formative assessment (an evaluation of learning in progress) and summative assessment (an evaluation of what has been learned) are well-established processes in GP education. Many of the Workplace-Based Assessment (WPBA) tools in the MRCGP have the effect of performing both of these functions simultaneously. This allows the trainer to assess previous learning and forms a useful framework for providing feedback to trainees on how they may improve their performance. You can find more details on the WPBA in Chapter 4, 'Succeeding at the MRCGP'.

Table 3.6

Using the curriculum to address training issues	
The training issue	**How to use the curriculum**
A doctor who is generally underperforming	• Evaluate the doctor's performance against the six areas of competence described in the core statement 1.0 *Being a General Practitioner* • Give constructive feedback • Think holistically – is there an external explanation for why the trainee is not performing well? • Identify learning needs and priorities • Use a spiral learning approach – start by focusing on the basic knowledge needs, then on applying the knowledge in practice, then on practising the more complex skills and finally on developing expertise
A doctor having difficulty with a specific competency or task	• Identify the competency (or everyday task) where the specific difficulty arises • Define the learning outcomes that together are required to perform that specific competency • Identify if the problem is related to a lack of knowledge or skill, or to an attitudinal issue • Plan targeted learning activities to address the specific outcome(s) identified
A doctor who is performing well and needs to be challenged further	• Review a topic-based curriculum statement in depth with the trainee • Observe how the specialty trainee adapts his or her generic skills to the specific context covered by the statement • Consider each of the core competences and essential application features in turn • Give constructive feedback • Identify further learning needs and priorities

A range of educational activities provides a platform for providing constructive feedback, including:

- random and problem case analysis
- case-based discussion tool (part of the WPBA)
- reviewing a learner's portfolio, logbooks or reflective diary
- video consultations (or listening in on phone consultations)
- joint/shared surgeries.

The Pendleton feedback rules[14] can be useful for formal feedback activities and are particularly helpful for those who are uncomfortable with giving or receiving feedback. It offers a useful model for people who tend to be overly self-critical as it forces them to describe what is positive about their behaviour or performance:

1 The learner performs the activity

2 Questions are allowed on points of clarification of fact

3 The learner describes what he or she did well

4 The person giving feedback says what he or she thought was done well

5 The learner describes what was not done so well and what could be done better

6 The person giving feedback says what he or she thought was not done so well and in a supportive manner suggests ways for improvement.

Table 3.7

Principles of constructive feedback

Principle	Example
Describe the behaviour you have observed rather than your own interpretation	'You didn't maintain eye contact with the patient and spoke in rather a flat tone', rather than 'You seemed bored and uninterested'
Describe specific examples	'You arrived late for your morning surgery on three occasions last week', rather than 'You're always turning up late for everything'
Remain non-judgemental	'It has been noticed that sometimes you don't reply when the reception staff say good morning', rather than 'The staff think you are rude and unfriendly'

Learning by teaching

Teaching can be an excellent way to learn – you never fully appreciate what you don't understand until you try to teach it to someone else! The need for GPs to develop teaching skills is reflected in the contextual statement 2.04 *Enhancing Professional Knowledge*. Many specialty trainees taking part in half-day release courses are involved in organising seminars and presentations for their peers as part of their learning programme.

Keeping up to date

As medical professionals, GPs are required (and are usually well motivated) to keep their knowledge and skills up to date and develop new skills as they are needed. This process is known as continuing professional development (CPD) and is an essential competency of modern general practice.

Some popular ways of keeping up to date are described in Table 3.8.

Table 3.8

Some popular ways of keeping up to date in general practice	
Review the journals	The *British Medical Journal* (BMJ) and the *British Journal of General Practice* (BJGP) contain news and articles of interest to GPs. The journal *Evidence-Based Medicine* contains evidence-based research reviews relevant to primary care. Many useful journals can be accessed online by RCGP members and Associates-in-Training free of charge at www.rcgp.org.uk
Essential Knowledge Updates	A six-monthly online update of new and changing knowledge relevant to general practice is available from the RCGP at: www.elearning.rcgp.org.uk
Read the GP press	The weekly GP papers include a lot of clinical information and produce a lot of free additional publications that contain information on recent developments in primary care
Journal watch	Several organisations, including the RCGP, offer an electronic journal watch service, which highlights and summarises the latest relevant research findings

Continued over

Courses and educational meetings	A number of courses offers GPs 'refreshers' on current topics of importance in general practice
Peer study groups	Many doctors find small study groups an invaluable way of sharing good practice and support. The RCGP First5 programme arranges groups for newly qualified GPs
Mailing lists	You can get on the email list of organisations such as the National Institute for Health and Clinical Excellence (NICE) (www.nice.org.uk) and the Scottish Intercollegiate Guidelines Network (SIGN) (www.sign.ac.uk), and receive regular updates free of charge

CPD has been defined as 'lifelong learning for all individuals and teams, enabling professionals to fulfil their potential while meeting the needs of patients and delivering the health outcomes and health care priorities of the NHS'.[15]

For a GP, this process involves taking time regularly to identify:

- personal learning needs

- practice development needs

- community and local health service needs.

GPs are required to provide evidence of their ongoing education, create learning plans and demonstrate how they are maintaining and improving their knowledge and skills during their annual appraisal. Once a year, every NHS GP must meet with a suitably trained appraiser to review his or her previous year's PDP and to agree new learning objectives for the following year (including GPs in training, although this is incorporated into the WPBA system). The underlying principle of appraisal is that professional development should be driven by individual needs and priorities.

Keeping a learning portfolio

Portfolio learning has become integrated into medical training. Foundation doctors are required to keep a portfolio as part of their training and all GP specialty trainees use the RCGP's web-based electronic portfolio (the Trainee ePortfolio), as part of the MRCGP assessment. The Trainee ePortfolio contains a PDP tool and, as it can transfer collected evidence of learning over to the Revalidation ePortfolio at the end of training, it forms an excellent base for a new GP to start building a personal learning portfolio that will grow during the rest of his or her professional career.

Portfolios are becoming increasingly popular in ongoing professional education too, and the RCGP now offers an ePortfolio to support revalidation. This enables a GP to document and reflect on significant professional events and educational activities, and to record and calculate the CPD credits they have earned towards the five-yearly revalidation of their licence to practise from the General Medical Council.

Reflection is a central part of portfolio-based learning, which involves the following steps:

- identifying your learning needs
- creating a PDP based on these needs (Table 3.9)
- using appropriate resources to meet these needs
- demonstrating what you have learned
- reflecting on the learning process and identifying new needs.

Table 3.9

A basic PDP template	
Learning need	To successfully manage the concerns of the mother of a child with glue ear and avoid an unnecessary referral
How this was identified	My referrals log and a letter from a local consultant indicate I am referring inappropriately to ENT
Educational activities	1 Read up on the natural history and management of glue ear in an ENT textbook 2 Tutorial planned on eliciting and addressing parental concerns with my trainer 3 Day at the local ENT clinic arranged
Time scale	Six weeks
Evidence of learning	1 My log shows I successfully reduced my referrals 2 Scored 87% in an ENT e-learning module 3 Positive feedback from trainer on video consultations

For detailed information on using the RCGP Trainee ePortfolio, see Chapter 4, 'Succeeding at the MRCGP'.

References

1 Kolb D A. *Experiential Learning: experience as the source of learning and development*. New Jersey: Prentice Hall, 1984.

2 Brookfield S D. *Understanding and Facilitating Adult Learning*. San Francisco: Jossey-Bass, 1986.

3 Knowles M S. *Andragogy in Action: applying modern principles of adult learning*. San Francisco: Jossey-Bass, 1984.

4 Middleton P, Field S J. *The GP Trainer's Handbook*. Oxford: Radcliffe Medical Press, 2001.

5 Schön D. *The Reflective Practitioner*. New York: Basic Books, 1983.

6 Schön D. *Educating the Reflective Practitioner*. San Francisco: Jossey-Bass, 1987.

7 Honey P, Mumford A. *Manual of Learning Styles*. London: P. Honey, 1982.

8 Briggs Myers I with Myers P. *Gifts Differing: understanding personality type*. Mountain View, CA: Davies-Black Publishing, 1995 [1980].

9 www.peterhoney.com [accessed May 2012].

10 *Rating Scales for Vocational Training in General Practice*. Occasional Paper 40. London: RCGP, 1989.

11 Eve R. Meeting educational needs in general practice – learning with PUNs and DENs. *Education for General Practice* 2000; **11**: 73–9.

12 Neighbour R. *The Inner Consultation*. Lancaster: MTP, 1987.

13 Tuckman B, Jensen M. Stages of small group development. *Group and Organizational Studies* 1977; **2**: 419–27.

14 Pendleton D, Schofield T, Tate P, *et al*. *The Consultation: an approach to teaching and learning*. Oxford: Oxford Medical Publications, 1984.

15 NHS Executive. *Continuing Professional Development: quality in the new NHS*. Leeds: NHS Executive, 1999.

4 Succeeding at the MRCGP

The MRCGP assessments

Since 2007, it has been compulsory for every doctor undertaking a GP training programme in the UK to successfully complete the MRCGP assessment.

The current MRCGP assessment has three components:

1 **Applied Knowledge Test** – a multiple-choice question test, performed on computer

2 **Clinical Skills Assessment** – an OSCE-style assessment of GP consulting skills

3 **Workplace-Based Assessment** – a continuous portfolio-based assessment of skills, attitudes and behaviours demonstrated in the workplace.

This chapter describes what the three components involve, which skills and attributes they assess – and how to complete them successfully.

The MRCGP – a very brief history

The *MRCGP examination* was born in 1965 and became compulsory for newly qualified GPs seeking entry into membership of the College in 1968. Since then, it has developed as the discipline of general practice has developed and assessment methodologies have become more sophisticated. The changing examination has reflected advances in clinical practice, the growing expectations of patients and the changing role of the GP.

Summative assessment was introduced for all GP trainees completing their training in September 1996. This was the first introduction of a national assessment package for general practice and one of the biggest changes in vocational training in the United Kingdom. Its most important function was to identify incompetent doctors and therefore to protect patients from harm.

Summative assessment was a test of *minimal* competency in the wide range of knowledge, skills and attitudes required of an independent GP – there was evidence that the system that preceded summative assessment did not effectively identify incompetent doctors,[1] and the public wanted reassurance that only doctors who had achieved an agreed minimum standard of competence should be able to enter the profession. The vast majority of GP trainees had no difficulty in passing summative assessment and increasing numbers began to take the MRCGP examination to prove that they had reached a high, rather than a minimum, standard.

Over time, as most doctors opted to take the MRCGP exam, the two assessments grew closer together, until summative assessment was replaced by the 'new' MRCGP in 2007.

Development of the current MRCGP assessments

While the new curriculum for GP training was being developed, the RCGP also started to work on its partner, the 'new' MRCGP assessment, which was designed to test the contents of the curriculum. These were both introduced in August 2007, following approval by the Postgraduate Medical Education and Training Board (PMETB),[i] the relevant body at the time.

The current MRCGP involves a combination of Workplace-Based Assessment (WPBA), which covers the whole three years of GP training, and two formal examinations – the Clinical Skills Assessment (CSA) and the Applied Knowledge Test (AKT). The standards for all the components of the MRCGP, which is the GP licensing qualification, are set by the RCGP (and approved by the GMC). The assessments themselves are delivered partly by the College and partly in partnership with local deaneries, the regional bodies responsible for organising GP training.

The MRCGP competency areas

The MRCGP assessments are designed to assess GP trainees against the RCGP curriculum, to ensure they are competent for independent practice. The 12 competency areas assessed in the WPBA are set out as shown on Table 4.1. The required *standard* expected of the doctor is described in 'word pictures' within the full version of the competency framework (available at www. rcgp.org.uk).

These competency areas are not only tested in the WPBA. For example the knowledge base for areas 3, 4, 5 and 6 are tested in the AKT. Communication, decision making and interpersonal skills are also tested in the CSA (see Table 4.7, on p. 51). It is important, therefore, to realise that the competency areas are not a 'soft touch' that can be skimmed over. The majority of the skills, attitudes and behaviours described in the WPBA competency framework are also tested in the formal AKT and CSA examinations.

i PMETB has since been abolished and its functions have been taken over by the General Medical Council (GMC).

Table 4.1

The 12 MRCGP competency areas

The MRCGP WPBA assessments have been designed around 12 competency areas which represent the important aspects of general practice that can be appropriately assessed:

1 Communication and consultation skills

This includes how a GP communicates with patients and uses recognised consultation models and communication techniques

2 Practising holistically

This considers the ability of the doctor to operate in physical, psychological, socioeconomic and cultural dimensions, taking into account feelings as well as thoughts

3 Data gathering and interpretation

This involves gathering and using data for making clinical judgements, the choice of physical examinations and investigations, and how they are interpreted

4 Making a diagnosis/making decisions

This examines how a GP adopts a structured, conscious approach to decision making

5 Clinical management

This assesses how a doctor recognises and manages common medical conditions in primary care

6 Managing medical complexity and promoting health

This looks at the aspects of care that go beyond managing straightforward problems, including the management of co-morbidity, uncertainty, risk and approaches to health rather than just illness

7 Primary care administration and IM&T

This includes the appropriate use of primary care administration systems, effective record keeping and information technology for the benefit of patient care

8 Working with colleagues and in teams

GPs must be able to work effectively with other health professionals to ensure good patient care, including the sharing of information with colleagues

9 Community orientation

This involves managing the health and social care of the practice population and local community

Continued over

10 Maintaining performance, learning and teaching
This looks at how doctors maintain their performance and ensure effective continuing professional development of themselves and others

11 Maintaining an ethical approach to practice
This examines how GPs ensure they practise ethically, with integrity and a respect for diversity

12 Fitness to practise
The GP's awareness of when his or her own performance, conduct or health, or that of others, might put patients at risk and the actions taken to protect patients

How the MRCGP assessments relate to the curriculum

The curriculum describes the core knowledge, skills and attitudes required to be a competent GP. However, measuring all these qualities in a way that is accurate, reliable and valid is not a straightforward task. It is not easy, for example, to directly measure a GP trainee's true *attitudes* towards a patient – to do so would require considerable mind-reading skill, which is an ability that few GP trainers possess.[ii]

Deeper features, such as attitudes, can be assessed indirectly, however – because, although they may seem inaccessible, they show themselves through the *behaviours* that result. To give a couple of examples, a rigid attitude to patient care may show itself as being dogmatic and not sharing decisions. A lack of commitment to self-improvement may be seen through not completing assignments on time. These important professional attitudes, just like the knowledge and skills, need to be learnt and discussed, which is why they need to be described in the curriculum.

Because behaviours are explicit and can be seen and assessed, the 12 MRCGP competency areas focus on the behaviours a GP performs in the workplace. These behaviours are based directly on the six areas of competence and the three essential application features described in the core curriculum statement (See Chapter 5, 'The core curriculum'). The relationship between the curriculum and the MRCGP competency areas is shown in Table 4.2.

The role of the clinical and educational supervisors

During GP specialty training, each trainee receives both educational and clinical supervision.[2] Each of these roles performs different educational functions.

---

ii Although many of them can do a good job of convincing you otherwise.

Table 4.2

The curriculum and the new MRCGP assessments

The RCGP curriculum	The MRCGP assessments
The curriculum describes the knowledge, skills, attitudes and expertise required to be a GP	The assessments have been designed to test the key behaviours that can be reliably assessed but are not designed to represent the entirety of general practice on their own
The curriculum	**Related MRCGP competency areas**
Primary care management	Clinical management
	Working with colleagues and in teams
	Primary care administration and IM&T
Person-centred care	Communication and consultation skills
Specific problem-solving skills	Data gathering and interpretation
	Making a diagnosis/making decisions
A comprehensive approach	Managing medical complexity and promoting health
Community orientation	Community orientation
A holistic approach	Practising holistically
Contextual features	Community orientation*
Attitudinal features	Maintaining an ethical approach to practice
	Fitness to practise
Scientific features	Maintaining performance, learning and teaching

* The MRCGP 'community' orientation competency assesses both the community orientation area of the curriculum and the contextual features of the doctor.

The *educational supervisor* is responsible for the overall supervision and management of a specified trainee's educational progress during a training programme. The educational supervisor is responsible for carrying out the trainee's six-monthly reviews. In most training programmes, the role is usually carried out by a GP trainer.

Each trainee should also have a named *clinical supervisor* for each placement in their hospital-, practice- and community-based posts. A clinical supervisor is a senior clinician responsible for overseeing a trainee's clinical work and providing constructive feedback during his or her training placement. The clinical supervisor must complete the Clinical Supervisor's Report (CSR) towards the end of each placement.

Sometimes these two supervisory roles may be performed by the same person. For example, during practice-based placements, the GP trainer usually carries out the role of educational and clinical supervisor simultaneously.

Getting to grips with the MRCGP

The current MRCGP assessments are considerably more detailed and sophisticated than their predecessors and involve many acronyms. To help you get to grips with these, you may find it useful to refer to our *MRCGP acronym-buster* on Table 4.3.

Table 4.3

The MRCGP acronym-buster!

The MRCGP suffers from an epidemic of TFLAs – three- and four-letter acronyms. Here is what some of the commonly used acronyms stand for:

AKT	Applied Knowledge Test
CbD	Case-based discussion
CEX	Clinical evaluation exercise
COT	Consultation observation tool
CSA	Clinical Skills Assessment
CSR	Clinical Supervisor's Report
DOPS	Direct observation of procedural skills
EMQ	Extended matching question
MCQ	Multiple-choice question
MSF	Multi-source feedback
OSCE	Objective structured clinical examination
PSQ	Patient satisfaction questionnaire
RITA	Record of in-training assessment
SBA	Single best answer questions
WPBA	Workplace-Based Assessment

The Applied Knowledge Test

The Applied Knowledge Test (AKT) is a multiple-choice question test, which is delivered and marked by computer. There are 200 items in the test, which must be completed in three hours. There are four main types of questions:

1 *Extended matching questions*

Each question consists of a scenario that has to be matched to an answer from a list of possible options. There may be several possible answers but you must choose only the most likely answer from the list of options. This may represent the single most likely diagnosis or the single most appropriate statement that matches the scenario.

Box 4.1

An example of the extended matching question style *iii*
Option list • Eczema. • Psoriasis. • Herpes simplex. • Scabies. • *Molluscum contagiosum.* • Cutaneous larva migrans.
Instruction For each patient described below, select the **SINGLE MOST LIKEY** diagnosis. Each option may be used once, more than once, or not at all.
Items • A 45-year-old man presents with thickened red plaques with a silvery scale on the extensor surfaces of his knees and elbows. • A 5-year-old girl has developed a small cluster of umbilicated pearly papules on her chest, but is otherwise well. • A 19-year-old student attends with a widespread, excoriated rash on his arms, trunk and groin, which is intensely itchy, especially at night. Examination of his wrist reveals several small, irregular track-like marks.

iii The MCQ examples included here are intended to demonstrate the style of question and are not official new MRCGP exam questions.

2 *Single best answer questions*

This is a common multiple-choice question format. Each question consists of a statement or stem followed by a number of options, only one of which is correct.

Box 4.2

An example of a single best answer question style

Which is the **SINGLE MOST APPROPRIATE** first-line treatment for menorrhagia? **Select one option only**.

A   Mefenamic acid

B   The combined oral contraceptive pill

C   Endometrial ablation

D   Levonorgestrel-releasing intrauterine system

E   Hysterectomy

---

3 *Table/algorithm completion*

These questions are similar to the algorithm layout often found in guidelines that provide advice on management decisions. The candidate must select the answer that correctly completes the table, flowchart or algorithm. These will sometimes use the format of 'drag and drop' on the computer.

4 *Free-text questions*

These questions have recently been introduced to test areas of knowledge such as drug dosage calculations. The candidate is required to type in the answer, which will usually be a single word or a number. All of the answers in this format are manually scrutinised to allow for minor typographical variations.

New types of AKT questions

New types of questions are sometimes trialled as part of the development of the AKT, such as the use of audio-visual material. Any development is very carefully introduced and analysed to make sure it does not disadvantage candidates who are facing tests that their predecessors did not encounter.

Preparing for the Applied Knowledge Test

The AKT tests both clinical and non-clinical aspects of general practice knowledge and assesses the *application* of knowledge, including decision making, evaluation of evidence and undifferentiated problems, and decisions regarding patient safety. The questions are based on the knowledge contained within the RCGP curriculum and distributed as follows:

- clinical medicine (80%)

- administration and health informatics (10%)

- research, critical appraisal, evidence-based medicine and statistics (10%).

All questions address important issues relating to UK general practice and focus mainly on applied problem solving rather than simple recall of basic facts. The questions relate to current best practice rather than local arrangements and so should be answered based on published evidence – the AKT team has published a Content Guide to the AKT containing a list of relevant topics that might appear in the exam. Because some experience of real-life general practice is required, the AKT can only be taken during the ST2 stage of specialty training or later.

The AKT is offered three times a year at around 150 centres across the UK and trainees are able to attempt it up to three times in a 12-month training period. Trainees are limited to *four attempts* in total. For booking details, see the RCGP website (www.rcgp.org.uk). When you apply to take the AKT, there is a generic tutorial available on the website that you can review to familiarise yourself with the format of computer-based testing. On the day of the AKT, you will have a ten-minute tutorial with sample questions before starting the real exam. This will include an example of each of the question formats used in the test.

Questions are derived from accredited and referenced sources. These include review articles and original papers from well-known publications, including: the *British Medical Journal*, NICE and SIGN guidelines, the *British Journal of General Practice*, *Drugs and Therapeutics Bulletin* and the *Cochrane Review*. Questions on therapeutics and prescribing will be based on information from the *British National Formulary* and *BNF for Children*. Textbooks such as the Oxford Handbook series are used as the basis for many of the questions that are cross-referenced for reliability. Many of these journals and publications are available free of charge to RCGP members and Associates-in-Training via the RCGP website (www.rcgp.org.uk).

One of the best ways of preparing for the AKT is by ensuring you have a broad working knowledge of general practice, as described in the curriculum. At the end of each surgery, it can be helpful to jot down the topics you have encountered, and check what guidelines are available for these. The AKT covers common topics that are seen frequently such as asthma, but also rare but important topics such as meningitis. (We have extracted the core knowledge and skills from each of the curriculum statements in Chapter 6, 'The applied knowledge'.) Doing lots of practice MCQs can also be a highly effective way to prepare for the exam, although it is not the most inspiring way to learn general practice!

Table 4.4

Tips for preparing for the Applied Knowledge Test	
Practice MCQ questions	Practice MCQs to aid preparation are available both in books and online. There is a sample paper with 50 questions on the RCGP website (www.rcgp.org.uk)
e-Learning modules	RCGP Essential Knowledge Challenges (www.elearning. rcgp.org.uk), Doctors.net (www.doctors.net.uk) and BMJ Learning (www.bmjlearning.com) offer learning modules that contain MCQs and extended matching questions. GPnotebook (www.gpnotebook.co.uk) offers educational modules ('GEMS') on the key clinical topics that are useful for revision
Personal Education Planning (PEP) tool	RCGP Scotland's interactive e-learning resource includes MCQs mapped to GP curriculum topics [iv]
AKT Content Guide	A useful list of topics from the AKT team, detailing the knowledge base that might be tested in the AKT assessment (www.rcgp.org.uk)
Critical appraisal workbooks	Several books are available that offer data interpretation questions (e.g. interpreting ECGs, spirometry, audiometry)

The Clinical Skills Assessment

The Clinical Skills Assessment (CSA) is an assessment of a doctor's ability to integrate and apply clinical, professional, communication and practical skills appropriate for general practice. It takes the form of an OSCE-style examination with 13 stations, each lasting ten minutes. It is based on simulated consultations

iv Available at: www.elearning.rcgp.org.uk.

with specially trained actors playing the role of patients. Candidates undertake a mock 'surgery' and will remain at their station throughout the assessment while the simulated patients and examiners rotate around them.

How the CSA is marked

All the CSA examiners are fully trained and experienced MRCGP assessors. The examiner for each case marks every candidate on three areas – Data Gathering, Clinical Management and Interpersonal Skills. Each of these areas carries the same number of marks, which are added to create a final mark for that candidate.

As the mix of cases in the CSA exam varies from day to day (to prevent cheating), a new pass mark for the exam must be calculated every time. This involves a complex statistical process using the 'borderline group method'.[3] As well as marking the scores on the three areas described above, the examiners also separately rate the candidate overall – as a pass, a fail or a 'borderline'. This subjective rating does not affect that candidate's score, but is used to help calculate the overall pass mark for the day. The numerical marks of all the candidates placed in the borderline group for each case are then averaged. These averaged scores are then aggregated across all the 13 cases to create a 'cut score'. This score is then adjusted to take account of the standard error of measurement, resulting in the final pass mark!

Don't worry too much about how the pass mark is calculated. In a nutshell, the exam is carefully designed to pass those candidates who demonstrate that they are competent GPs and fail those that do not.

All candidates receive feedback on their performance.

Preparing for the CSA

The purpose of the CSA is to assess doctors' ability to bring together and apply their clinical, professional, communication and practical skills to a standard appropriate for general practice. For this reason, the CSA cannot be taken before the ST3 stage of GP training. It is held three times a year, during a three- or four-week period in February, May and November in a custom-made assessment centre. Trainees are limited to *four attempts* in total.

The CSA has been designed to focus on core GP skills that can be assessed outside the workplace to an agreed national standard (to reduce any distortion that might be introduced by individual trainer and local deanery variation).

Table 4.5

Aspects of general practice covered by the Clinical Skills Assessment	
Primary care management	Recognising and managing common medical conditions in primary care
Problem-solving skills	Gathering and using data for clinical judgement, choice of examination, investigations and their interpretation. Demonstration of a structured and flexible approach to decision making
Comprehensive approach	Demonstrating proficiency in the management of co-morbidity and risk
Person-centred approach	Communicating with patient and using recognised consultation techniques to promote a shared approach to managing problems
Attitudinal aspects	Practising ethically with respect for equality and diversity, with accepted professional codes of conduct
Clinical and practical skills	Demonstrating proficiency in performing physical examinations and using diagnostic and therapeutic instruments

Patient safety is also an important aspect of the CSA – one of the key functions is to identify potentially dangerous doctors. Examples of cases that might come up in the CSA include:

- communicating sensitively with a depressed patient (played by an actor) and assessing his or her suicide risk

- checking and demonstrating the inhaler technique of a patient with asthma

- identifying a mental health problem in a patient with a long-term physical condition

- demonstrating how to perform a targeted examination of a patient with hip pain or back pain.

Table 4.6

Tips for preparing for the Clinical Skills Assessment

360° feedback	Encourage colleagues to provide feedback on your management of patients – this can be useful when they subsequently see a patient you found challenging. What approach did they find successful?
Consultation analysis	Video lots of consultations and review them – use a variety of methods to analyse them. Watch videos with different GPs, your trainer or mentor, other GPs in the practice, your course organisers and your learning group (bearing in mind patient confidentiality and that you must obtain informed consent). Don't worry if you cringe at first when watching yourself consulting – this is entirely normal!
e-GP e-learning on physical examinations	The RCGP's CSA team have developed a series of e-learning sessions demonstrating some common GP scenarios and the physical examination skills you might be asked to demonstrate, available at: www.e-GP.org
Explaining diagnoses and treatments	Keep a list of all the diagnoses you make and treatments you recommend in a day. Practise explaining these to patients and ask for their feedback, so that you are skilled at doing this by the time you take the CSA
Learning groups	Learning groups are particularly suitable for preparing for the 'softer' topics, including ethical and professional dilemmas
Mock CSAs and revision courses	Some local training programmes may offer CSA practice stations and consultation scenarios. The higher-quality preparation courses for the MRCGP will include CSA practice stations
Role-play	Like sprouts at Christmas, role-play is one of those things you just have to do. It can be done with your peers, your trainer and other members of staff or even professional actors. Always bear in mind the rules of giving effective feedback and be sensitive until you are certain that everyone present is comfortable with giving and receiving feedback
Shared surgeries	Analyse a range of healthcare professionals' consulting styles (e.g. sit in, or watch a video they have made). What do they do well? What could they do better? You can learn lots from observing the tricks and techniques used successfully by other people. Also, ask a number of experienced GPs to observe you consulting and to provide you with feedback and advice. As the patients attending shared surgeries are largely unselected, this approach enables you to get immediate feedback on a whole range of consultation types

Continued over

Skills simulator laboratories	'Skills simulator labs' are useful for learning new procedures, especially those not performed in daily practice where gaining sufficient experience is otherwise difficult (e.g. minor surgical techniques, inserting catheters, Basic Life Support skills)

Doctors from different ethnic and professional cultures, or those who have difficulties communicating in English, may require additional targeted support during their GP training. This need can often become apparent when these doctors are preparing for the CSA, which requires doctors to not just understand scientific medicine, but also how it must be tailored to the socioeconomic status, educational level and broader understanding of the patient in the consultation.

For example, GPs have to learn how to think in a culturally tuned way to analyse evolving problems and manage changing risks; this goes beyond what protocols are capable of directing doctors to do. In some cases, although the doctor has a perfectly adequate grasp of language, it is the application of that language to social contexts (sociolinguistics) that makes the critical difference to the understanding between doctor and patient. It is also important that doctors learn not to consult in a 'formulaic' way, but to make their consultations feel natural and relaxed.

It is particularly important that any difficulties with thinking skills and communication skills, especially language, are identified and targeted as early as possible in training (e.g. in ST1). This enables the maximum amount of time for targeted training to be put in place and additional educational opportunities to be arranged.

A number of educational and supportive approaches can help trainees with language or cultural learning needs. These include starting peer study groups from the beginning of specialty training, ensuring that these remain small (e.g. three or four members) and, as people naturally tend to form groups with people of similar backgrounds to themselves, making sure that the groups are deliberately kept multicultural. This ensures that members of different cultures have opportunities to learn from each other and so develop the subtle skills required to communicate smoothly and effectively with people from different backgrounds.

The difference between passing and failing

Table 4.7 shows some of the characteristic behaviours demonstrated by candidates who pass and those who fail the CSA. It is based on a qualitative analysis carried out in 2009.[4]

Table 4.7

Behaviours of candidates who pass or fail the Clinical Skills Assessment

General features	• Fluent, interactive and relevant • Is able to take patient into medical world as a shared partner • Open about lack of knowledge or certainty and may use this constructively • Active monitoring during consultation	• Poor use of time • Uneasy with or unable to acknowledge own ignorance or uncertainty • More scripted summary than checking understanding • Unaware of personal space
Data gathering	• Can take a focused history that includes all relevant information • Embedding of questions in previous response	• Formulaic questioning that can become interrogative • Repetitive questioning • Sequence of questions does not make sense
Clinical management	• Appears knowledgeable and refers to recognised algorithms or modes of practice • Able to suggest solutions to problems or a range of reasonable management options likely to be agreeable to patient	• Insufficient knowledge base, or ability to think of realistic and effective alternatives • Fails to integrate and apply knowledge • Puts off making clinical decisions or a clear diagnosis • Doesn't appear to grasp the dilemma if there is one
Interpersonal skills	• Connects instantly with patient • Non-judgemental • Interested in the patient • Reformulates explanations using helpful metaphors • Can meet patient half-way – picks up patient's agenda, accent or cultural approach	• Doctor-centred/patient's concerns not addressed • Patronising • Unable to explain effectively – may be wrong or not tuned to patient • Inappropriate use of terms • Over patient-centred to the detriment of clinical outcome

Around 80% of candidates pass the CSA on their first attempt and only a small proportion need to take it more than twice.[5] Many trainees fail because they take the exam *too early* in their ST3 year. Trainees who fail the CSA should be offered extra support by their deanery to look into why this has occurred; it may be that certain factors in the trainee's learning environment need to be addressed or they are not consulting in a sufficiently patient-centred way, therefore failing to identify the nub of each case. Trainees should only apply to re-take the CSA when they and their educational supervisors are confident that they are ready to do so.

The Workplace-Based Assessment

The RCGP curriculum emphasises the importance of learning in the workplace and this importance is reflected in the Workplace-Based Assessment (WPBA) component of the MRCGP.[6]

The WPBA runs from the very start to the end of the training programme (i.e. ST1–3) and is designed to bring teaching, learning and assessment together into one continuing process; trainees gather evidence of their actual performance in the workplace regularly over time, which enables those aspects of professional behaviour that cannot be tested reliably by external examinations to be assessed (such as time management, communication and team-working).

Why is an assessment in the workplace needed?

There are many important attributes of a doctor that cannot be tested through traditional classroom-based exams or interviews. These include how we relate to our colleagues, how we take a role in making changes in the practice, and how we deal with errors and complaints on a day-to-day basis.

Importantly, the WPBA enhances the validity of the other MRCGP exams, because it tests essential skills, such as our diagnostic abilities, across a far wider range of clinical encounters than the ones we might face in a one-off examination. This ensures that very few skills are tested solely in one component of the MRCGP, which gives a more reliable 'global view' of each trainee's performance – a process known as triangulation – and this results in a fairer and more reliable system overall.

The assessment side of the WPBA

Evidence of performance is collected over all three years of training and recorded in a web-based portfolio (the RCGP Trainee ePortfolio).[v] This evidence is used to inform six-monthly reviews and, at the end of training, to make a holistic judgement about the fitness of the doctor for independent practice.

The evidence in the ePortfolio is organised in a structured framework, based on the 12 MRCGP competency areas (see section 5.1). This approach allows the educational supervisor to quickly judge the trainee's progress and give feedback in a systematic and comprehensive way.

The learning side of the Workplace-Based Assessment

Importantly, WPBA is an educational and developmental process as well as an assessment. It is intended to provide ongoing feedback to trainees throughout their training programme, to steer their learning and highlight areas of difficulty. This part of the process is led by the learner, who decides which items of evidence about learning he or she wishes to share with the clinical or educational supervisor.

The RCGP Trainee ePortfolio

The RCGP Trainee ePortfolio has been specially developed by the RCGP to enable every GP specialty trainee to collect all the evidence they need to complete WPBA. The ePortfolio stores the trainee's *Training Record*, which contains:

- **the evidence of competency** – the trainee's progress in the 12 MRCGP competency areas is recorded at regular intervals when the evidence of performance is regularly reviewed (see below)

- **a record of learning** – learning activities can be recorded (e.g. tutorials, group learning, seminars) and stored under the relevant curriculum statement heading

- **a technical skills log** – examination skills and procedures undertaken (e.g. joint injections, minor ops) can be recorded along with the direct observation of procedural skills (DOPS) assessment.

Collecting evidence in the ePortfolio

Much of the evidence used for the WPBA is intended to be collected and uploaded informally, through the use of templates that are completed by the trainee. In addition to this, a range of formal assessment tools (see below) have also been specially developed for gathering evidence both within the practice and externally. Some

v Available at: https://eportfolio.rcgp.org.uk.

of these tools are mandatory (i.e. every trainee must complete them at specified times during training) whereas others are optional.

Naturally occurring evidence

Much of the evidence of learning and performance is generated by the normal day-to-day activities a doctor carries out in the workplace. This is referred to as the 'naturally occurring' evidence. For example, a GP trainee might consult with a patient with poorly controlled diabetes, then do a search for studies on improving patients' concordance with diabetes management, review and present these to a practice meeting, and apply this learning when the trainee follows up the patient. All of this learning activity can be recorded in the learning log of the ePortfolio and would count towards WPBA.

A range of templates has been developed in the ePortfolio to enable different types of learning activity to be recorded. These include:

- Audit/Projects

- Clinical Encounters

- Courses/Certificates

- eLearning Sessions

- Lectures/Seminars

- Out-of-Hours Session

- Professional Conversations

- Reading

- Significant Event Analysis

- Tutorials.

You can also upload attachments to support the entry you have written (e.g. certificates, documents, audits, presentations, etc.).[vi] If the activity resulted in a further learning need remember to record this too and you can link this to your Personal Development Plan (PDP).

Although the naturally occurring evidence is collected and recorded informally by the trainee, it must be linked to the relevant area(s) of the curriculum and shared with the clinical or

---

vi You can even attach copies of the 'Thank You' cards you receive from your more grateful patients! (However, be sure these are anonymised first.)

educational supervisor for it to count in WPBA; the supervisor then comments and validates the entry against one or more of the 12 MRCGP competency areas.

Each entry in the learning log must be linked to the area(s) of the curriculum to which it relates. For example, if you create an entry about caring for a terminally ill patient, you might link this to clinical statement 3.09 *End-of-Life Care*.

Many trainees try to link their learning log entries to too many areas of the curriculum. However, your educational supervisor (and the panel of assessors) will be interested in the *quality* of the entries that you have made, rather than the *quantity*, as long as you have entered a reasonable number for each curriculum area for your stage of training and show a comprehensive spread of curriculum coverage at your final review in ST3. This means you need to learn how to write good learning log entries!

Writing high-quality learning log entries

According to the RCGP's WPBA standards group, a high-quality learning log entry should show:[7]

- some evidence of critical thinking and analysis, describing your own thought processes

- some self-awareness, demonstrating openness and honesty about your performance and some consideration of feelings generated

- some evidence of learning, appropriately describing what needs to be learnt, why and how

- appropriate linkage to the curriculum

- demonstration of behaviour that allows linkage to one or more MRCGP competency areas.

Table 4.8 (overleaf) shows some of the features that suggest different degrees of reflection in a learning log entry. Review some of your recent entries and assess them against these criteria.

Formal Workplace-Based Assessment tools

The WPBA occurs throughout the entire three-year GP training period. To support this, the ePortfolio has been designed to work with a number of formal tools that must be used by every GP trainee at certain points during his or her training programme. This is in order to collect specific types of evidence about performance.

Table 4.8

Framework for evaluating the reflective entries in your ePortfolio[7]

	Not acceptable	Acceptable	Excellent
Nature of information provided	Entirely descriptive, e.g. lists of learning events/certificates of attendance with no evidence of reflection	Limited use of other sources of information to put the event into context	Uses a range of sources to clarify thoughts and feelings. Demonstrates well-developed analysis and critical thinking, e.g. using the evidence base to justify or change behaviour
Demonstration of critical analysis	No evidence of analysis (i.e. an attempt to make sense of thoughts, perceptions and emotions)	Some evidence of critical thinking and analysis, describing own thought processes	Shows insight, seeing performance in relation to what might be expected of GPs
Demonstration of self-awareness	No evidence of self-awareness	Some self-awareness, demonstrating openness and honesty about performance and some consideration of feelings generated	Consideration of the thoughts and feelings of others as well as him or herself
Evidence of learning	No evidence of learning (i.e. clarification of what needs to be learnt and why)	Some evidence of learning, appropriately describing what needs to be learnt, why and how	Good evidence of learning, with critical assessment, prioritisation and planning of learning

Tools used in secondary care

To review progress during hospital posts, trainees undergo six-monthly reviews with their secondary care clinical supervisor (e.g. a consultant) and their educational supervisor. During this process, the trainee's clinical supervisor completes a Clinical Supervisor's Report (CSR). Reviews carried out in secondary care make use of the following validated tools.

Direct observation of procedural skills (DOPS)

This is a tool for assessing the GP trainee's technical skills in relevant clinical procedures. This tool can be used in primary care if there are skills that have not already been signed off during the secondary care placements. However, trainees are encouraged to maximise the opportunity to have the required DOPS procedures assessed in secondary care.

Mini-clinical evaluation exercise (mini-CEX)

This is a validated case-based discussion tool and is used in place of the consultation observation tool (COT) while the GP trainee is working in secondary care. It is modelled and adapted from the mini-CEX used in the Foundation Programme.

Tools used in primary care

During the primary care placements, the following assessment tools are used. It is *mandatory* to use these and they are designed for use *within the practice*.

Case-based discussion (CbD)

This is a structured interview designed to assess the trainee's clinical and professional judgement across a range of cases selected for discussion.

Consultation observation tool (COT)

This is a tool designed to help supervisors assess videoed or observed consultations, and to give feedback to trainees on developing communication and consultation skills for independent practice. It is adapted from the old MRCGP video examination criteria. It is used in primary care in place of the mini-CEX.

Patient satisfaction questionnaire (PSQ)

This is designed to collect and evaluate feedback from patients.

Tools used in both primary and secondary care

The following assessment tool is used in both the primary and secondary care placements and is externally moderated:

Multi-source feedback (MSF)

This is a web-based tool designed to collect and evaluate feedback from peers and colleagues

Table 4.9

Tools for collecting evidence for the Workplace-Based Assessment[8]

MRCGP competency area	MSF	PSQ	COT	CbD	CEX	CSR
Communication and consultation skills	✓	✓	✓		✓	✓
Practising holistically		✓	✓	✓		✓
Data gathering and interpretation	✓		✓	✓	✓	✓
Making a diagnosis/making decisions	✓		✓	✓	✓	✓
Clinical management	✓		✓	✓	✓	✓
Managing medical complexity and promoting health				✓	✓	✓
Primary care administration and IM&T				✓		
Working with colleagues and in teams	✓			✓		✓
Community orientation				✓		✓
Maintaining performance, learning and teaching	✓				✓	✓
Maintaining an ethical approach to practice	✓			✓		✓
Fitness to practise	✓			✓		✓

A number of additional *optional* assessment tools have been designed for the supervisor and trainee to use to gather evidence of performance. It is not compulsory to use all the tools available but trainees will need to make sufficient use of them to enable the collection of enough evidence to complete the various parts of the WPBA:

- videos of consultations

- practice audit

- Significant Event Analysis

- referrals and prescribing analysis.

Direct observation of procedural skills (DOPS)

The DOPS tool is designed to assess how a trainee performs some of the procedures and examination skills common to general practice. For the purposes of GP training, some of the procedures are mandatory and others are optional.

Most of the DOPS procedures will be observed during secondary care attachments, although they can be done at any appropriate point in the training programme; the trainee is responsible for choosing the timing and the observer. The observers may be experienced hospital specialty registrars, staff grades, consultants or appropriately skilled nurse practitioners – the key principle is that the observer has to be well-skilled and properly trained in the procedure they are watching you do. Asking fellow trainees to act as your DOPS observer is not allowed!

There are eight mandatory procedures, for which every trainee must be successfully recorded as competent by the end of GP training. You will have to complete all of these under observation during your GP specialty training period in order to complete the DOPS requirements, even if you have previously performed them during your Foundation posts. The procedures are:

- application of a simple dressing

- breast examination

- cervical cytology sample taking

- female genital examination

- male genital examination

- prostate examination

- rectal examination (may be combined with prostate examination)
- testing for blood glucose.

There are also a number of recommended but optional procedures that, if undertaken, can be recorded in the ePortfolio using the DOPS tool. These optional procedures may change from time to time but at the time of publication include:

- aspiration of effusion
- cauterisation
- cryotherapy
- curettage/shave excision
- excision of skin lesions
- incision and drainage of abscess
- joint and periarticular injections
- hormone replacement implants
- proctoscopy
- suturing of a skin wound
- taking skin surface specimens for mycology.

When planning a DOPS, allow time for discussion and feedback on the procedure from your observer – it is intended to be an educational exercise as well as an assessment. Also, ask the observer to justify his or her rating of you in the feedback comments by giving some specific examples of good or poor technique and explaining how you might improve. To help guide observers and trainees, some deaneries have produced guidance on appropriate standards for some of the procedures and examinations.[vii]

In addition to the technical skills, the DOPS form requires the observer to rate other important aspects, such as respect for the patient's dignity, communication throughout the procedure, obtaining of consent, and following hygiene procedures. For this reason, the procedures need to be performed on real patients in a real clinical setting.

vii For examples, see www.bradfordvts.co.uk.

Mini-clinical evaluation exercise (mini-CEX)

A mini-clinical evaluation exercise (mini-CEX) is a short summary of a doctor–patient interaction that occurs within a secondary care setting, such as a hospital. It is designed to assess the trainee's clinical skills, behaviours and attitudes.

A mini-CEX takes about 15 minutes to complete and may be observed by the clinical supervisor or the educational supervisor. It may also be observed by experienced specialty registrars, staff grades, consultants and nurse practitioners. Feedback is provided immediately by the observer and the evidence is rated and recorded in a simple template in the Trainee ePortfolio. Following feedback from the observer, a brief plan for future learning and development should be drawn up.

Each mini-CEX should illustrate a different clinical problem and the trainee is expected to select a range of different clinical topics and patient groups, to create a balanced picture of progress. During ST1 and ST2, each full-time trainee will be expected to undertake six observed encounters per year (three before each six-monthly review). If in primary care, the mini-CEX is replaced by the COT.

Case-based discussion (CbD)

For a full-time trainee in ST1 and ST2, a minimum of six CbDs should be carried out per year (three before each six-monthly review) and twelve CbDs in ST3 (six before the six-monthly review and six before the final review).

The trainee is responsible for requesting the CbD, selecting the cases and making sure that the documentation is properly completed for each one. He or she should select two cases for each CbD and present copies of the relevant records to the clinical supervisor or educational supervisor at least one week before the discussion. One case will then be chosen for discussion.

Guidance on the sort of cases that a trainee should consider and the areas to be explored should be given by those conducting the CbD (particularly in the early stages of training).

Having an effective discussion

A CbD is a structured interview between a trainee and an educator. It is principally a test of clinical and non-clinical reasoning that aims to explore the doctor's thinking, insight and justification for decisions – especially the decisions around management that are made in the consultation. This makes it one of the most important assessments in the MRCGP.

CbD is used in both primary and secondary care settings, so a CbD might be carried out by your educational supervisor or a clinical supervisor, depending on circumstances. Although all 12 MRCGP competency areas may be explored in a CbD, some are more apparent because they are central to professional judgement. Behaviours that relate to the doctor's ability to 'understand', 'recognise' or 'consider' are particularly relevant.

From the educator's perspective, questions in a CbD should be based on the presenting problem, using this as a jumping off point to explore what the doctor thought (or did not think) about this and reflecting on *why* he or she reasoned in this manner. It is important to maintain focus on a few key areas and increase the challenge to help determine the trainee's standard of reasoning in any particular area. Attempting to cover too many competency areas at once can result in an unfocused discussion that fails to test decision making to the appropriate degree and makes it harder to give specific feedback to help the trainee improve.

The focus and degree of challenge in a CbD will depend on the insight and experience of the trainee and his or her stage of training. Earlier in training, the discussion may concentrate on clinical management and decision making, ensuring safe practice. It may also explore other areas like holism and working with colleagues. During these early stages of training, the trainee will not have had much experience with dealing with complex problems, such as co-morbidity or managing health care in the community. But at the later stages of training the CbD can usefully explore the trainee's understanding of complexity and community orientation. This does not mean that these more challenging aspects cannot be explored at earlier stages of training; indeed, this can help trainees to develop an understanding of the basics of these important concepts. It's just that the main objective earlier in training should be on getting a good grounding, tested through CbD, of the areas in which the trainee has had some experience.

Because the MRCGP competency framework is unfamiliar territory to most trainees, especially in early training, it is important for the supervisor to give guidance as to what sort of cases it may be useful to explore. This will help the trainee to select relevant material to bring for assessment and thereby help him or her to understand the MRCGP competency framework. It is important to cover a range of different topics but also different *contexts* of care (e.g. outpatients, GP consultations, home visits and out of hours). Don't select 'easy' cases as these will not reveal the more complex skills that need to be demonstrated.

An assessment needs to be made at the end of the focused discussion. Assessors should then use the outcomes of their assessment to give the trainee specific feedback, teaching formatively on the aspects of the case discussed and signposting to further learning opportunities. This gives the trainee greater insight into the process and enables him or her to select relevant material for the next CbD or assessment. In this way, CbD becomes a teaching tool that is valued by those completing it, rather than just an assessment tool with no apparent relevance to education.

After the discussion, the educator uses a structured template to record the CbD in the Trainee ePortfolio, mapping the evidence against the relevant MRCGP competency areas – it can be helpful for trainees to suggest which of the areas they feel their management of the case demonstrates. Descriptions of what determines 'insufficient evidence', 'needs further development', 'competent' and 'excellent' for each competency area are listed in the Trainee ePortfolio.

More information and resources about the CbD process and discussion/feedback cycle can be found at www.wpba4gps.co.uk under 'Training/Case Based Discussion'.

Consultation observation tool (COT)

A consultation observation tool (COT) is an assessment of the trainee's consultation skills carried out in the primary care setting. The exercise can be carried out in two ways: a trainee might record a number of consultations on video and select one for assessment or, alternatively, arrange in advance for his or her supervisor to directly observe a consultation. The selected consultation should be reviewed and discussed by the trainee and supervisor together. The trainee's performance is then rated by the supervisor in the Trainee ePortfolio, using the MRCGP competency areas and a set of COT criteria (see Appendix 2).

The aim of the COT is for the supervisor to observe the trainee's consultation and other clinical skills in action, leading to feedback and discussion about areas for further improvement. More complex consultations will generate more feedback and discussion, and so lead to greater improvements over time.

As with CbD, consultations for the COT should be chosen from a range of topics and patient contexts. In all cases, the patients must give their written consent.

Over the entire time spent in general practice, the trainee must include at least one case from each of the following categories of patient:

- a child (aged 10 or under)

- an older adult (aged over 75 years)

- a patient with a mental health problem.

In each of the ST1 and ST2 stages, a full-time trainee must undertake a minimum of six COTs (or mini-CEX, if in secondary care), ensuring there are three available before each six-monthly review. In ST3, a trainee must do 12 COTs (six before the six-monthly review and six before the final review).

Box 4.3

Don't be scared of recording your mistakes!

Videoing and reviewing your consultations is one of the most effective ways to improve your consultation skills. It is a good idea to plan a regular surgery session each week for videoing; this allows for the reception team to check with patients who book in advance that they are willing to be videoed, and for the required equipment, consent forms and explanatory information to be made available.

Reviewing your consultations on screen can be nerve-wracking at first, especially when watching them with your peers, but this feeling will ease with time. It is important to remember that the COTs you record in your ePortfolio that do not rate well against some MRCGP competency areas won't count against you in the MRCGP[viii] – as long as by the end of training you have enough positive evidence to show competence in all the core areas. In fact, difficult consultations can be used very effectively in the ePortfolio as evidence to demonstrate your learning and the resultant improvement in your skills over time.

Using a structured approach, such as the COT or another consultation framework, can help provide focused feedback. This, combined with the wisdom of an experienced GP who can suggest alternative approaches, is an invaluable way of learning.

Videoing your consultations may also reveal aspects of your consulting style that you did not previously know about. For example, it is how one of the authors of this book discovered they had a distracting tendency to slide around the room on their office chair during consultations (which looked especially comical on *fast forward*), a problem quickly fixed by removing the casters from the legs of the chair. . . .

viii Unless you do something outrageous, dangerous or illegal, of course – a general rule that applies to all doctors throughout their careers!

Patient satisfaction questionnaire (PSQ)

The Patient Satisfaction Questionnaire (PSQ) gives patients an opportunity to score the trainee's performance, in particular their view of the doctor–patient relationship and the degree of empathy shown during a consultation. This feedback helps the trainee and supervisor identify attitudes and skills that may need further development.

There is a standard procedure that must be followed for the PSQ. First, the trainee and educational supervisor agree a start date and a date for the feedback interview. On the start date, the questionnaires and letters of explanation are handed by the receptionist to consecutive patients consulting with the trainee (even if the patient is unlikely to respond). The receptionist and trainer must complete a declaration form, stating they have followed the procedure, and return this to the deanery.

The patient completes the questionnaire after the consultation and hands this back to the receptionist. This process continues until 40 completed questionnaires have been returned, which might take a few days. These questionnaires are then forwarded to the deanery, which processes them and enters the results into the Trainee ePortfolio.

At first, the results are only visible to the educational supervisor, who reviews them and makes them available to the trainee (and his or her GP trainer, if this trainer is not their educational supervisor). Results are anonymised and include the mean, median and range for each question. These data are worth reviewing, in case the mean score has been skewed by a small number of particularly harsh or overly generous responses.

The feedback interview should be arranged for a period when there is plenty of time for discussion and there will be no interruptions. To be effective, the person giving the feedback (e.g. the educational supervisor) will need to use his or her skills to help ensure the advice is non-judgemental, specific and helpful to the trainee. [ix] Remember to record the discussion in the learning log, using the 'Professional Conversation' template and to add any action points to the PDP.

During ST3, when the trainee is in primary care, the PSQ should be completed once during months 31 to 34. It may also need to be completed in ST1 or ST2, if the trainee is working in a primary care placement (see Table 4.10 on p. 71 for the timetable).

More information on the PSQ, including the questionnaire itself, can be found on the RCGP website (www.rcgp.org.uk).

---

ix Saying 'the patients think that you're a really rubbish doctor' is an example of poor feedback technique.

Multi-source feedback (MSF)

The multi-source feedback (MSF) tool allows a range of colleagues to give their views on the clinical performance and professional behaviour of the trainee. It provides useful information that can be used for reflection and self-evaluation, and to guide future development.

The trainee should arrange a date for the MSF and a follow-up date to meet and discuss the feedback with his or her educational supervisor (or GP trainer, if this is not the same person). As with the PSQ, the feedback meeting should be arranged at a time when there will be no other distractions or interruptions.

Two MSFs must be completed in ST1 and a further two in ST3. When completing the MSF during a secondary care placement, the trainee must select five clinicians, each with different job titles. During a primary care placement, the trainee selects five clinicians (i.e. GPs and practice nurses) plus five non-clinicians (e.g. receptionist, secretary, practice manager, etc.). All the respondents must have observed the trainee in the workplace.

The trainee must give the invited respondents a standard instruction letter; this explains the process and the closing date for submitting their feedback. Depending on local arrangements, the educational supervisor (or GP trainer, if different) will need to be briefed by the trainee on which team members have been invited to complete the MSF.

The process for completing the MSF forms is managed online:

- respondents log onto the Trainee ePortfolio, giving their name and GMC number of the trainee. They can then enter their feedback comments into the MSF form. Non-clinicians answer just the first question, while clinicians answer both questions

- the educational supervisor must check with a sample of respondents that they did indeed complete the MSF, although their individual responses will remain anonymised.[x]

On the closing date, the results are sent to the trainee's educational supervisor – these are the free-text comments and the breakdown of scores. There will also be data on the mean, median and range of scores. Once the educational supervisor has reviewed them, the results will be available within the Trainee ePortfolio and visible to the trainee.

As with the PSQ, the person giving the feedback (e.g. educational supervisor) will need to ensure the discussion is supportive

---

x Any trainees who attempt to cheat by filling in the MSF forms themselves risk referral to the GMC – so don't do that!

and helpful to the trainee. Record the discussion in the ePortfolio learning log, using the 'Professional Conversation' template and add any action points to the PDP.

Other Workplace-Based Assessment requirements to record in the ePortfolio

Cardio-pulmonary resuscitation (CPR) training

In order to complete the MRCGP, each trainee must demonstrate that he or she is competent in cardio-pulmonary resuscitation (CPR) and automated external defibrillation (AED). The best way to do this is to upload a valid certificate of competency in CPR & AED in the learning log of the Trainee ePortfolio, so this can be validated by your educational supervisor.

To be valid, the training must take place during GP specialty training and must conform to the Resuscitation Council (UK) Guidelines in place at the time. The certificate needs to be issued by a Resuscitation Council (UK) advanced life support (ALS) instructor or equivalent. Basic resuscitation training is an NHS requirement too, so many practices will arrange regular approved training, in which you should participate.

Out-of-hours experience

'Out-of-hours' (OOH) care is the primary care work undertaken between 18.30–08.00 on weekdays and all day at weekends and public holidays. In 2004, the responsibility for providing care at these times was transferred from general practices to NHS primary care organisations. As a result, the majority of general practices no longer provide OOH care for their registered patients – instead, this care is provided by a different primary care service, known as an OOH care provider.

As gaining the Certificate of Completion of Training (CCT) at the end of GP training licenses that doctor to work unsupervised in any capacity in UK general practice, including for an OOH care provider, GP trainees must be trained in OOH work.

Trainees are responsible for organising their sessions with their local OOH care provider and for making sure that they complete the required number of hours. It is sensible to book your sessions at the start of each general practice placement and to ensure they are evenly spread out. A variety of sessions is recommended (e.g. including overnights and weekends). Some OOH providers now operate an online booking system that allows trainees to book shifts directly.

Trainees should record all of their OOH sessions in the learning log of the ePortfolio, using the 'out-of-hours' template. All OOH sessions should be shared and discussed with the educational supervisor, so they can be validated. Sometimes, a trainee's OOH clinical supervisor is not his or her educational supervisor, in which case the clinical supervisor will need to complete an OOH session feedback sheet. The trainee must then share this feedback sheet with the educational supervisor as evidence of his or her attendance.

Towards the end of the training programme, the trainee's educational supervisor will check that the required number of OOH sessions have been completed. The current minimum recommendation is that a trainee should do the equivalent of one session (of 4–6 hours) per month while working in general practice, spread evenly over the course of the training programme. So if you are doing 18 months in general practice, you will need to do at least 18 OOH sessions. However, some deaneries may adjust the minimum requirement to take into account local circumstances.

It is important not just to document the hours spent on-call but also to document evidence of learning and performance (e.g. reflections on cases you have managed, significant events, feedback from colleagues, etc.). Remember that many of the other educational and assessment tools in the ePortfolio can be applied to OOH contacts with patients – for example, if your evidence of OOH competence is weak, you may find it helpful to arrange a case-based discussion (CbD) with your clinical or educational supervisor on a patient you saw in an OOH setting.

Clinical Supervisor's Report (CSR)

Towards the end of each secondary care post, the clinical supervisor writes a short, structured report on the trainee. This considers the trainee's:

- knowledge base relevant to the post
- practical skills relevant to the post
- the professional competencies of the trainee.

The Trainee ePortfolio contains an online CSR form for clinical supervisors to complete, with definitions of the competencies to make writing it easier. Although it is the clinical supervisor's responsibility to write the report, our experience suggests that trainees may need to give their supervisors some gentle encour-

---

xi A pointy stick may be required for some busy consultants.

agement at the appropriate time,[xi] as the report needs to be completed before each six-monthly meeting with the educational supervisor takes place. It also helps supervisors if trainees complete their learning logs regularly, rather than suddenly releasing a large number of entries a short time before a report is due. The supervisor needs to use the learning log entries as evidence for some of the decisions made in his or her report.

When writing and discussing the report, both clinical supervisors and trainees may find it helpful to refer to Chapter 5, 'The core curriculum', and Chapter 6, 'The applied knowledge', as well as Appendix 1, to remind themselves of the GP knowledge and skills most relevant to that particular training placement.[xii]

The purpose of the CSR is to highlight any significant developmental needs identified during a placement, as well as to identify strengths. The focus of the report should be on the trainee's progress in terms of the evidence of competency that he or she has demonstrated, rather than making a pass or fail judgement.

The information in the CSR will be considered at the six-monthly review with the educational supervisor, when a decision will be taken as to whether the trainee's progress is satisfactory – or whether any additional training might be required.

The six-monthly review

At six-month intervals, every specialty trainee meets with his or her educational supervisor (and his or her clinical supervisor while in secondary care) to undertake an interim review of progress and current performance. The ePortfolio evidence that the trainee has collected to date is reviewed, a self-assessment completed and the trainee's progress evaluated by the educational supervisor in each of the 12 MRCGP competency areas. A learning plan will then be agreed, with all the information being recorded in a standardised format in the Trainee ePortfolio.

The six-monthly review process takes 1–2 hours and involves:

- reviewing the evidence of achievement in the ePortfolio (including any Clinical Supervisor's Reports, if in secondary care)

- making a judgement of performance

- giving feedback

- setting educational goals and objectives

- planning the next phase of training.

xii The RCGP has developed a 20-minute e-learning session for clinical supervisors on the CSR, available at: www.e-GP.org.

The reviews provide a valuable opportunity to look at the breadth of coverage of the curriculum and identify gaps, which will affect preparation for the AKT and CSA.

Throughout the entire training period, the standard against which each trainee is judged is *always* the level of competency expected of a doctor who is certified to practise independently as a GP. In other words, from the very start of training, trainees are always judged against the standard they should have reached at the end of training.

Obviously, this means that if you are in your first two years of training, you are very unlikely to meet this high standard and your educational supervisor will identify developmental needs in lots of the MRCGP competency areas – this is exactly what the WPBA process is meant to do, so that you can plan your future training around your areas of greatest need.

After you have had each six-monthly review, remember to update the PDP in the Trainee ePortfolio.

Annual Review of Competence Progression (ARCP)

The Annual Review of Competence Progression (ARCP) process is the formal review and assessment of every GP trainee that takes place during each year of specialty training at deanery level.[xiii] It is run by a panel of experts, including clinicians and a lay representative, who are responsible for approving each trainee's progress from one specialty training year to the next. Deaneries are responsible for ensuring that all GP specialty trainees are assessed by the ARCP panel at least once a year.

If the panel receives good reports about a trainee from the educational and clinical supervisors and the ePortfolio demonstrates that he or she is making the required progress, then the panel review will take place 'virtually' and they will approve the trainee without the need for a face-to-face meeting. It is therefore very important that trainees make sure they have the required evidence available in their ePortfolio by the ARCP panel's review deadline.

The minimum evidence required in the ePortfolio before each ARCP review is:

1 **Assessments:** the required set of assessments for the year about to be completed, as shown in Table 4.10, must be uploaded before the ARCP panel's submission deadline. These should show evidence of competency appropriate to the stage of training and demonstrate improvements over time

---

xiii For more information on ARCP panels, see the 'Gold Guide', available at www.mmc.nhs.uk.

Table 4.10

Timetable showing the required evidence for the Workplace-Based Assessment (for a full-time GP trainee)		
Specialty Training Year 1	**Specialty Training Year 2**	**Specialty Training Year 3**
For the six-month review:	*For the 18-month review:*	*For the 30-month review (in primary care):*
• 3 × COT or mini-CEX	• 3 × COT or mini-CEX	• 6 × CbD
• 3 × CbD	• 3 × CbD	• 6 × COT
• 1 × MSF	• PSQ,* if not completed in ST1	• 1 × MSF
• DOPS*	• DOPS**	
• CSR*	• CSR**	
* if in secondary care	* only if in primary care ** if in secondary care	
For the 12-month review:	*For the 24-month review:*	*For the 34-month review:*
• 3 × COT or mini-CEX	• 3 × COT or mini-CEX	• 6 × CbD
• 3 × CbD	• 3 × CbD	• 6 × COT
• 1 × MSF	• PSQ,* if not completed in ST1	• 1 × MSF
• 1 × PSQ*	• DOPS**	• 1 × PSQ
• DOPS**	• CSR**	
• CSR**		
* only if in primary care ** if in secondary care	* only if in primary care ** if in secondary care	

Notes:

- COT is used in primary care and mini-CEX in secondary care

- DOPS can be completed in both primary and secondary care, when an appropriate opportunity arises. It is not repeated once the mandatory practical skills have been assessed as satisfactory

- patient satisfaction is assessed only in primary care

- MSF involves clinicians only when in secondary care and both clinicians and non-clinicians in primary care.

2 **Learning log:** this should contain evidence of learning in a range of different contexts (e.g. inpatients, outpatients, consultations, home visits, OOH) and should demonstrate an appropriately broad coverage of the curriculum. Remember that the ARCP panel can only see the entries that have been shared and validated by the educational supervisor. While there is no required minimum number of learning log entries required for each staged review, there should be a sufficient number of quality entries to provide evidence of learning during each review period. A good benchmark for trainees is to complete one or two reflective learning log entries per working week. Remember it is important to provide a balanced portfolio of evidence, so as to present a range of learning log entries, including clinical encounters, personal and supervised learning

3 **PDP:** this should be up to date and contain SMART learning objectives, a plan to meet them, and evidence that previously identified objectives have been met. It is important to set learning objectives for each training placement within the review period and to 'close the learning loop' by checking your progress against each of these objectives before your review with your educational supervisor

4 **Educational supervisor's and clinical supervisor's reports:** the arrangements in each deanery may vary, so check the local arrangements.

Any trainees making unsatisfactory progress will be referred for a face-to-face ARCP panel review at the deanery. This is not always because the trainee is failing – those who are training 'Less Than Full Time', or returning from maternity leave or extended sick leave, will also need to be reviewed on an individual basis.

Before each ARCP panel review, the educational supervisor completes a report. This must be reviewed and accepted by the trainee in order for it to be considered by the ARCP. If the educational supervisor has concerns, he or she may recommend a panel review.

If a panel review is requested, or the ePortfolio contains unsatisfactory or missing evidence, the trainee will be required to attend in person. The ARCP panel will first review and discuss the trainee's ePortfolio evidence without the trainee being present. The trainee will then be invited to discuss the outcome once the panel has made a decision and may explain any mitigating circumstances. The outcomes of ARCP panel meetings are now recorded entirely in the Trainee ePortfolio.

If the ARCP panel decides not to recommend the trainee for progress to the next specialty training year, the deanery will make arrangements for additional training with the trainee, depending on his or her individual circumstances.

The final review

Shortly before the end of the three-year training period, a final summative review is carried out. At this point, the educational supervisor makes an overall recommendation to his or her local deanery regarding the readiness of the specialty trainee for independent practice.

To complete training successfully, the trainee's ePortfolio must demonstrate evidence of proficiency in all 12 of the MRCGP competency areas. Failure to reach the required standard triggers a review by the ARCP panel, which then judges whether the WPBA has been completed satisfactorily. As the WPBA involves the evaluation of a trainee's progress over three years of training it cannot be completed early and will only be signed off towards the end of the training programme.

The final ARCP panel, held near the end of the third year, decides whether to recommend to the RCGP that each trainee be awarded a CCT for general practice. This final recommendation requires evidence that the trainee has covered the curriculum, successfully completed all the required WPBAs, passed the AKT and the CSA, and received satisfactory reports from his or her educational and clinical supervisors.

Once the successful trainee has received his or her membership of the RCGP and CCT, and been added to the GMC's GP register, he or she is entitled to practise independently as a GP – and then the *really* hard work begins!

References

1 Campbell LM, Murray TS. Summative assessment of vocational trainees: results of a 3-year study. *British Journal of General Practice* 1996; **46**: 441–4.

2 *A Reference Guide for Postgraduate Specialty Training in the UK* ('The Gold Guide 2010'), www.mmc.nhs.uk/pdf/Gold%20Guide%202010%20Fourth%20Edition%20v08.pdf [accessed May 2012].

3 Downing SM, Tekian A, Yudkowsky R. Procedures for establishing defensible absolute passing scores on performance examinations in health professions education. *Teaching and Learning in Medicine* 2006; **18**: 50–7.

4   Rendel S, Hawthorne K, Roberts C. General comments about features/ behaviours observed in passing and failing candidates in the CSA, www.rcgp.org.uk/gp-training-and-exams/mrcgp-exam-overview/~/media/ Files/GP-training-and-exams/General-comments-about-features-behaviours. ashx [accessed May 2012].

5   MRCGP Annual Report 2010. www.rcgp.org.uk/gp-training-and-exams/ mrcgp-exam-overview/mrcgp-annual-reports.aspx [accessed November 2012].

6   Swanwick T, Williams N, Evans A. Workplace assessment for the licensing of general practitioners: a qualitative pilot study of a competency-based trainer's report. *Education for Primary Care* 2006; **17**: 5.

7   RCGP WPBA Standards Group. Hallmarks of good practice in information recording in the ePortfolio, wwww.primarycare.severndeanery.nhs.uk/ training/curriculum/annual-review-of-competence-progression-arcp/guide-to-arcp-panels-2012/ [accessed November 2012].

8   Royal College of General Practitioners. WPBA tools, www.rcgp.org.uk/ gp-training-and-exams/mrcgp-workplace-based-assessment-wpba. aspx [accessed November 2012].

Part II

The condensed curriculum

In the following sections of the book, we condense the curriculum to a fraction of its original size. We have done this by distilling the key educational content and separating it into two simple components – *the core curriculum* and *the applied knowledge*.

The core curriculum

This section of the book explains the core knowledge, skills, attitudes and expertise a doctor needs in order to be a competent GP. It is based on the RCGP's core curriculum statement 1.0 *Being a General Practitioner*.

The applied knowledge

This section of the book explains how to learn and apply the core knowledge and skills in everyday general practice. It includes some practical tips for learning them and some useful educational resources. It builds on the contextual statements and clinical examples described in the RCGP curriculum.

The condensed curriculum is not meant to replace the full RCGP curriculum, but rather to help you understand its key messages and important educational content. Our aim is to make the curriculum easily accessible to all GP learners and teachers, and to enable readers to gain an overall understanding of how to learn and teach the core knowledge and skills that are central to good general practice.

5 The core curriculum

The core of general practice

The first RCGP curriculum statement, *Being a General Practitioner*, is the heart of the curriculum. It describes the core knowledge, skills, attitudes and expertise a doctor needs in order to be a competent GP.

These core items of knowledge and skill are grouped into 'areas of competence', which provide a broad framework that helps you to learn general practice. This chapter explains these six areas of competence and gives some suggestions on how to learn them.

How the areas of competence were identified

Before the first version of the curriculum was created, several documents had been written that defined the *generic* competencies of a doctor. These generic competencies are the professional abilities and attributes that are expected of every doctor, regardless of his or her specialty. In addition, the curriculum describes areas that are *specific* to performing as a GP, based on the framework for general practice produced by WONCA Europe.[1]

The publication *Good Medical Practice*,[2] produced by the General Medical Council (GMC), provides a framework for judging the performance of all doctors. The RCGP and the General Practitioners Committee of the British Medical Association have used this as the basis for a document more specific to general practice, *Good Medical Practice for General Practitioners*.[3] The RCGP curriculum has been mapped to this document to make sure all of the generic professional competencies have been covered.

This language used in the curriculum has changed since the first edition of this book – what were previously known as core competences are now known as 'areas of competence'. The phrasing of the learning outcomes within each competence has also changed to a more personalised style (e.g. changing from 'the patient' in the old version to 'your patient' in the revised version).

A quick overview of the areas of competence

The first three areas of competence focus mainly on the GP consultation:

1 Primary care management

This is about managing your contacts with patients in primary care. It includes addressing people's unselected problems, co-ordinating care with other primary care professionals and with specialists, providing appropriate care to patients in the practice and making effective use of the health service.

2 Person-centred care

This involves being able to establish an effective doctor–patient relationship that demonstrates respect for the patient's autonomy, an ability to set priorities and act in partnership with patients, providing continuity of care and coordinating care.

3 Specific problem-solving skills

As generalists, GPs need to adopt a problem-based approach rather than a disease-based approach to their patients. This requires a number of specific skills, including selective history taking and physical examination and targeted investigations; making diagnoses related to the incidence and prevalence of conditions in the community; and formulating an appropriate and effective management plan. GPs deal with conditions that present early on in the course of an illness and in an undifferentiated way, so you need to become familiar with using appropriate GP techniques such as 'time as a diagnostic tool', 'incremental investigation' and 'tolerating uncertainty', spotting conditions or symptoms that may be serious and intervening urgently when required.

The remaining three areas of competence are more subtle and complex. Some may consider them as representing the 'woolly' aspects of general practice. They involve taking a wider perspective than just the immediate issues arising in the consultation:

4 A comprehensive approach

This involves mastering the skills to simultaneously manage multiple complaints and pathologies in one individual, managing both acute and chronic health problems that may coexist, successfully promoting health and implementing disease prevention strategies.

5 Community orientation

This requires the ability to reconcile the health needs of individual patients and the health needs of the community in which they live, taking account of the resources that are available. This requires consideration of the GP's responsibilities more broadly than the consulting room: to include the practice population, the local community and the wider health service.

6 A holistic approach

This involves caring for the whole person in the context of the patient's values, his or her family beliefs, family system, and culture in the larger community. It also involves the consideration of a range of therapies based on the evidence of their benefits and cost. An understanding of our own limitations as GPs is essential because of the emphasis on the therapeutic partnership between GP and patient.

Our tips for learning and teaching the areas of competence

The following pages describe the six areas of competence of general practice in detail. Each area of competence has a number of more detailed learning outcomes.

With each learning outcome we have included relevant tips and suggestions for interpreting, learning or teaching that outcome. These tips are drawn from a variety of sources including the published literature, educational workshops, the advice of established trainers, course organisers, programme directors and other GP educationalists. The authors are all working GPs involved in education and have borrowed heavily from their own practical experience of learning, teaching, training and caring for patients in everyday general practice.

The six areas of competence

Competence 1 – primary care management

This is about dealing competently with any and all of the problems with which your patients may present.

As family doctors, GPs work in the community, where the population has a lower prevalence of serious disease. It is crucial, therefore, that GPs understand concepts of health, function and quality of life, as well as disease. GPs play an important role in disease prevention and health promotion, risk management, chronic disease management, and in palliative and terminal care. They also need to be conscious of healthcare costs and understand the concept of cost-efficiency.

Primary care involves working with a team of health professionals, both within the practice and in the local community, and also working with specialists in secondary care, so every GP must learn to integrate different disciplines within the complex team of the NHS. GPs must also learn the importance of supporting patients' decisions about the management of their health problems and communicating how their care will be delivered. GPs also have a role to play in improving the quality of their local services, with growing responsibilities for population health and commissioning.

1.1 Managing primary contact with patients and dealing with unselected problems

This means that, as a GP, you should:

1.1.1	Understand the epidemiology of problems presenting in primary care
Our tips	A GP should be familiar with how patients present in the early stages of illness and develop a good sense of which conditions are common and which conditions are rare and/or potentially serious. Similarly, a GP must be aware of red-flag symptoms and signs that may indicate a potentially serious condition. A GP must also understand important risk factors and how these influence decisions on investigation and management.

Here are some ways to learn about epidemiology in primary care:

- review Chapter 6, 'The applied knowledge', which contains the common clinical conditions with which you should become familiar

- find information about disease prevalence at different practices and in different areas of the country from the Quality and Outcomes Framework (QOF) prevalence data, available at the NHS Information Centre (www.qof.ic.nhs.uk)

- review epidemiological information published by reputable bodies (e.g. Cancer Research UK publishes cancer statistics at www.cancerresearchuk.org).

1.1.2	**Master an approach that allows easy access for patients with unselected problems**
Our tips	Patients rarely walk in saying, 'Doctor, I have a pulmonary embolism.' Rather, they present with a collection of symptoms or concerns that may or may not fit familiar patterns. GPs must therefore develop a consulting style that enables them to rationalise unselected complaints and formulate an understanding of the key issues. This will include developing skills in eliciting information and active listening in order to obtain the relevant information, and summarising skills to check your understanding of the patient's ideas, concerns and expectations. GPs also need the ability to apply their medical knowledge appropriately to make sense of the patient's narrative.
	GPs who are particularly good at consulting tend to develop a flexible consulting style, adopting a range of approaches and techniques that can be put to use when needed, depending on the context of the consultation and the preferences of the individual patient.
	For tips on how to develop your consultation skills, see contextual statement 2.01 *The GP Consultation in Practice* in Chapter 6, 'The applied knowledge'.

1.1.3	**Use an organisational approach to the management of chronic conditions**
Our tips	In many practices, chronic disease management is carried out in nurse-led clinics, as opposed to routine GP surgeries. GPs need to develop the appropriate skills not only to manage individual patients' chronic diseases on a one-to-one basis but also to organise chronic disease care within their practice and to work effectively with primary care and secondary care colleagues.

Continued over

Ways to learn about the organisation of chronic disease management include:

- finding out how chronic disease management is organised in your practice and in the practices of your GP colleagues – there is a surprising amount of variation between practices

- looking into how these practices develop and maintain their chronic disease registers. What processes do they have for recalling patients for chronic disease reviews?

- attending or running a chronic disease management clinic

- reviewing your practice's protocols and computer templates. (What does an annual diabetes or asthma check actually involve?)

- auditing practice chronic disease outcomes against recognised standards

- reviewing QOF targets and your practice's achievement data

- discussing with the practice manager or nursing team leader about how a particular clinic was set up and the issues encountered

- reviewing your practice's chronic disease registers and identifying individual cases where you could become involved

- obtaining feedback from patients who attend the clinics.

1.1.4	**Know the conditions encountered in primary care and their treatment**
Our tips	There is a massive amount of knowledge for a GP to potentially assimilate, as general practice is the broadest field of medicine. It is essential to learn how to identify what knowledge you do or do not need to learn in order to perform competently.
	The knowledge contained within the curriculum statements describes much of the knowledge with which every GP should be familiar. (We have condensed this in Chapter 6, 'The applied knowledge'.) This forms a good basis for general practice although is not all encompassing; the knowledge you will require for life as a GP continually evolves over time and will depend on your individual circumstances.
	Here are some popular methods of identifying learning needs in general practice:

- keeping a log of learning needs arising from patients you see – a log is especially useful at the start of GP training when you want to remember to look up lots of straightforward pieces of information

- PUNs and DENs[4]

- the Johari window[5]

- random and selected case analysis

- confidence and competency rating scales

- formative assessments

- clinical questions logbook

- practice exam questions and MCQs

- referring to the curriculum areas of competence and the MRCGP competency areas.

Once you have identified your learning needs you need to formulate a system for recording them and your action plans – this can form the basis of your Personal Development Plan (PDP). Both the RCGP Trainee and Revalidation ePortfolios contain tools to help you do this. Resources that support learning and provide information for specific clinical areas are described in the relevant parts of Chapter 6, 'The applied knowledge'.

1.2 Cover the full range of health conditions

This means that, as a GP, you should:

1.2.1	**Know the preventive activities you need for the practice of primary care**
Our tips	'Prevention is better than cure' – or at least it saves some of the work. Find out what preventive activities the practice participates in already (e.g. smoking cessation, men's/women's/teenage health clinics, sexual health screening, cancer screening programmes). Is there any preventive activity important to the local population that the practice should be participating in but currently isn't?

1.2.2	**Develop the skills you need in acute, chronic, preventive, palliative and emergency care**
Our tips	As a generalist you must develop the skills required to deal with every problem that comes through the door – patients might arrive as 'worried well', 'ill but not too sick', 'very sick' or even 'moribund' – and a competent GP must be able to react appropriately and implement appropriate initial management.

Continued over

GPs in hospital training may find that it is hard for them to gain enough experience to feel comfortable about managing certain groups of patients by the time they start work in primary care. However, all hospital jobs should bring opportunities to develop both specific and general skills that will be useful in future life as a GP. Some hospital jobs (e.g. acute medicine, emergency medicine) provide good urgent care experience, while others may provide a range of chronic disease experience (e.g. old-age medicine, community hospital jobs).

If you are working in a hospital-based placement, consider what opportunities exist in your current post for you to gain useful experience and which 'gaps' in experience you may wish to focus on later, in primary care. See Appendix 1 of this book for practical tips on how to make the most of your secondary care posts.

1.2.3	Develop the clinical skills you need in history taking, physical examination and the use of ancillary tests for diagnosis
Our tips	Focused history and examination skills are key to being an effective GP – especially in the primary care context where time is short and access to diagnostic tests is often limited. A GP needs to be able to elicit sufficient useful information to diagnose conditions rapidly and accurately, assess their severity and decide whether further investigations are indicated. The Clinical Skills Assessment (CSA) of the MRCGP tests this important competency.
	Joint surgeries (preferably with a variety of experienced practitioners) are a good way of picking up useful consulting tips, gaining feedback on current performance and for bringing back complex patients for a more experienced opinion.

1.2.4	Develop the skills you need in therapeutics, including drug and non-drug approaches to treatment
Our tips	As a GP you need to become familiar with the repertoire of frequently used treatments (both drug and non-drug) and their indications, contraindications and common or potentially serious side effects.
	Evidence-based practice is central to this learning outcome and you should monitor the evidence for the therapeutic interventions you initiate on an ongoing basis. As a working GP, you may quickly become comfortable with a select group of 'favourite' treatments, which should mean you are

very familiar with their use. This includes knowledge of risks and benefits (which is a good thing). However, on the negative side, it may make you reluctant to use less familiar treatments that may have been shown to be superior, or alternatively may make you reluctant to stop using treatments that are no longer recommended.

A number of publications and information sources are available to aid treatment decisions. These include the *British National Formulary* (BNF), the *Drugs and Therapeutics Bulletin* and the BMJ's *Clinical Evidence*, which provide information about the evidence around therapeutics.

Your Primary Care Trust (PCT) will also issue local prescribing guidelines and your practice may have its own protocols and formulary.

1.2.5	**Be able to prioritise problems**
Our tips	There is a limit to how many things you can manage at one time – this applies both to the multiple problems of an individual patient and to the individual problems of multiple patients! Not forgetting your own non-clinical problems too!

When consulting, it is often helpful to encourage a patient to briefly 'unpack' all of his or her problems at the start (when it will often become apparent that they are all linked to one underlying issue). You should then discuss which problems it would be best to concentrate on, given the time available, and which may be more appropriate to discuss at another time.

One useful technique for prioritising multiple problems is to categorise them into *urgent* or *non-urgent* and then into *serious* or *less serious*. The urgent and serious problems should be addressed first, the urgent but less serious problems should be dealt with next, the non-urgent but serious problems should be addressed properly at the appropriate time, and the non-urgent, less serious problems can be deferred until time permits (with appropriate safety-netting – as per Neighbour's five-checkpoint consultation model).[6] Obviously, the GP's and patient's view of what is urgent and what is serious may differ, and this is where good negotiation skills are required!

1.3 Coordinate care with other professionals in primary care and with other specialists

This means that, as a GP, you should:

1.3.1	**Know how NHS primary care is organised**
Our tips	Near the start of your placement, find out who works in your practice and what their roles are. Ideally, this should be covered during an induction programme. Pay particular attention to non-clinical members of the team as you are likely to be less familiar with their roles. Next, find out about who is involved in the wider primary care team that has direct contact with the practice (e.g. district nurses, health visitors, midwives, counsellors, physiotherapists).
	Then there is a range of wider health professionals who work in the community (e.g. podiatrists, opticians, community pharmacists, specialist nurses, visiting consultants) and whose roles vary from locality to locality.
	Your local NHS commissioning organisation will be able to provide you with up-to-date information on the primary care services available in your area. Information is also available through the 'Choose and Book' system.
	GPs are about to be thrust into the centre of a massive restructuring of how primary care is delivered. At the time of writing probably the best place to get up-to-date information on this is the RCGP.

1.3.2	**Understand the importance of excellent communication with patients and staff for effective teamwork**
Our tips	The ability to work as an effective team player and team leader is essential to general practice. Even singlehanded GPs must work effectively on a daily basis with other healthcare professionals. At the heart of teamwork is good communication and an appreciation for the abilities of others. The multi-source feedback (MSF) assessment, required for both the MRCGP and for revalidation, aims to help you improve your team-working skills.

1.3.3	**Be able to work as a team member and team leader in providing services to patients**
Our tips	There is much evidence in the literature that the leadership attitudes and skills of clinicians are critical promoters (or barriers, if they are lacking) to the development of functioning and effective multidisciplinary healthcare teams.[7]

To develop these attitudes and skills, doctors need sufficient time and opportunity to take responsibility for their patients' care. There should be focus during this time on the development of the skills required to communicate freely and clearly with professionals from a range of disciplines across health and social care boundaries. Belbin has described nine different team roles (www.belbin.com)[8] that can provide insights into how individuals function within teams – and why some teams may work more effectively than others.

To improve the services they provide patients, GPs need to learn how to collate, interpret and act on feedback within their teams covering the whole pathway of care experienced by the patient – i.e. not just episodic, individual feedback but continuous, whole-system feedback.

1.4 Master effective and appropriate provision of care and health service utilisation

This means that, as a GP, you should:

1.4.1   Know the structure of the healthcare system and the function of primary care within the wider NHS

Our tips

The NHS is an ever-changing and increasingly complex organisation! Find out who is the most politically astute GP in the practice; he or she may be well placed to tell you all about the latest NHS reforms, future threats and opportunities, and the impact of political developments on your practice.

Arrange a tutorial with your practice manager to discuss these issues and other organisational developments, such as service redesign and commissioning.[9]

Other useful contacts include your Local Medical Committee (LMC) and clinically led commissioning group representatives. Your course organiser may be able to arrange one of these to resource a seminar on NHS structures and organisations.

- The weekly GP newspapers, the BMA website (www.bma.org.uk) and the RCGP website (www.rcgp.org.uk) contain lots of information on NHS changes affecting primary care.

1.4.2	**Understand the processes of referral into secondary care and other care pathways**

Our tips	It is essential for GPs to be able to access appropriate ongoing care for their patients. There is currently a major shift towards the provision of specialist care 'closer to home' in the community. Also, the concept of 'patient care pathways', which describe how a patient receives care over time in both primary and secondary care sectors, has influenced how services are now designed.[10]
	Practice secretaries and administrators are often a great source of useful knowledge and have a great deal of experience in how the local health services and referral systems work. Some practices will keep a folder, intranet or database containing local referral information. The 'Choose and Book' system also contains information on local NHS services. It is also important to become familiar with the key national referral initiatives (e.g. the two-week wait) and your local hospitals' referral guidelines.
	The RCGP online course 'Improving Patient Journeys' explores the process of referral and how you can improve the quality of your referrals (available at www.elearning.rcgp.org.uk).

1.4.3	**Manage the interface between primary and secondary care, including unscheduled care and communication with other professionals**

Our tips	The 'interface' refers to the various points of contact that occur between primary and secondary care. Managing this interface involves a number of skills. These include maintaining good continuity of care, ensuring effective communication between health professionals (to hand over, share and take back clinical responsibility), dealing appropriately with patient demand for access to services and managing unrealistic patient expectations.
	Maintaining a log of your referrals or carrying out an audit of your interactions with secondary care will help to identify aspects that work well and areas for improvement. Problems arising around the interface between primary and secondary care can often be the cause of adverse events (e.g. delayed referrals, failure to act on recommendations from secondary care).[11] These are often highly suitable incidents for a Significant Event Audit (SEA).

1.4.4	**Participate in service management and service improvement**

Our tips   GPs are taking on greater responsibility to improve and re-design the services in their local area. The increased complexity of providing high-quality care to an ageing population, combined with the increasing need to bring care 'closer to home', means that health care and social services must become more integrated and tailored to the needs of local populations. GPs, as family doctors based in the community, are central to this process.

In England, the responsibility of GPs extends further than in the other home nations and includes the commissioning of local services. Commissioning is the process of assessing the needs of a population, planning, procuring and monitoring services for that population, and then monitoring and evaluating the impact of those services. To perform this task, GPs, public representatives and other professionals work together in commissioning groups. They do this with local authorities, service providers (e.g. hospital trusts) and a range of third-sector organisations.

All practices in England will have a local lead for commissioning; contact the commissioning team to find out what is happening in your area and consider attending meetings of your local commissioning group.

1.5 Make available to your patients the appropriate services within the healthcare system

This means that, as a GP, you should:

1.5.1	**Develop your communication skills for counselling, teaching and treating patients and their families/carers**

Our tips   Communication skills are central to the discipline of general practice – after all, GPs spend most of their working day talking to people.

Theory: read up on the main consultation models (see the contextual statement 2.01 in Chapter 6) and counselling models (e.g. neurolinguistic programming [NLP], problem solving, cognitive behavioural therapy [CBT]).

Practice: observing how other doctors consult, joint surgeries, videoing consultations (all with appropriate feedback and reflection) and patient feedback are great ways to improve communication skills. You could also consider going on a consultation skills course if you have identified specific areas for improvement.

1.5.2	**Develop your organisational skills for record keeping, information management, teamwork, running a practice and auditing the quality of care**
Our tips	As a trainee you should be encouraged to get involved in the practice's business and clinical organisational meetings as these offer valuable practical experience of the nuts and bolt of running a practice. Try and complete at least one full audit cycle during your time in primary care. Evidence of participation in regular audit is also a mandatory requirement for five-yearly revalidation.
	These individual skills are covered in more detail in the contextual statements 2.01–2.04, explored in Chapter 6, 'The applied knowledge'. There is also a useful RCGP e-learning course on record keeping in general practice, available at www.elearning.rcgp.org.uk.

1.6 Act as an advocate for the patient

This means that, as a GP, you should:

1.6.1	**Develop and maintain a relationship and style of communication that does not patronise but treats your patients as equals**
Our tips	Many GPs identify strongly with the role of patient advocate and see steering their patients successfully through the health system, in order to obtain the best possible outcome, as one of their most important tasks.[12]
	This is about much more than adopting an approachable style when communicating with patients in a consultation, although that aspect is of utmost importance. It is also about the steps you take to actively involve patients in making decisions and how effectively you are able to share your power as a doctor, so that even your most vulnerable patients are sufficiently enabled and supported to make those decisions.
	Outside the consulting room, this competency relates to how you involve patients in decisions about the practice (e.g. when considering changes to the appointments system). Beyond the practice, it relates to how you engage with the public, including the disenfranchised, when gathering views and making decisions about service improvement, re-design and commissioning.

| 1.6.2 | **Show effective leadership, negotiation and compromise** |

Our tips

GPs fulfil a number of other important roles in the NHS; in particular they are responsible for the health of their local population and for managing the use of limited health resources. This 'gatekeeper' role means it is not always possible for a GP to act exclusively in the sole interest of one individual patient without disadvantaging another. Because of this, tensions can arise in the consultation and negotiation, and compromise is often called for. GPs must balance their role of patient advocate with their other responsibilities to the wider NHS while maintaining an effective and equitable relationship with their patients.

As well as relating to patients, this competency also applies to dealings with other professionals (e.g. colleagues, secondary care, Primary Care Organisations, etc.). This can be a good topic to explore in a group learning activity. Practice managers can often pass on handy tips about how they deal with difficult GPs!

Competence 2 – person-centred care

Being 'person-centred' is a way of thinking and acting that considers the patient as a unique person in his or her own unique context, taking into account the patient's preferences and expectations at every step in the consultation.[13] It is based on the concepts of autonomy, human rights, choice and social inclusion, and is now considered a fundamental part of good medical practice. In large part this approach has been driven by changes in Western society, culture and political values, but there is also a large body of evidence that a person-centred approach results in higher patient satisfaction and better health outcomes.[14]

2.1 Adopt a person-centred approach in dealing with your patients and their problems, in the context of the patients' circumstances

This means that, as a GP, you should:

2.1.1	Use your basic scientific knowledge in understanding the individual, together with his or her aims and expectations in life
Our tips	In addition to direct contact with patients, other strategies for gaining an understanding of the individual patient include reviewing the patient's notes for the observations of colleagues; relevant social issues and previous decisions about care the patient has made; visiting the patient at home; considering the other family members who are registered with the practice; and discussion with other professionals involved in the patient's care.

2.1.2	Develop a frame of reference to understand and deal with the family, community, social and cultural dimensions of a person's attitudes, values and beliefs
Our tips	Patient narratives can provide the GP with an individually tailored framework for approaching a patient's problems holistically, and can help to identify a patient's preferred management options.
	Narrative-based medicine [15] is concerned with how patients construct stories out of life events, which they may or may not relate to their health. Narratives also offer a framework for addressing non-biopsychosocial qualities of health and disease such as spiritual and moral issues, which may form part of people's illnesses but are not covered by traditional health and illness models.

2.1.3	**Master patient illness, sickness and disease concepts**

Our tips   Helman's 'folk model of illness'[16] and the 'health belief model'[17] are easy to understand. These models attempt to explain patient views of health and disease, and the patient's resultant behaviour. However, they have been criticised for making the assumption that patient decisions are always predominantly rational and failing to take into account the role emotions may play in patients' decisions about their illnesses. Other models of health and disease that have been developed include biomedical, psychosomatic, humanistic, existential and transpersonal.[18]

2.1.4	**Apply these skills and attitudes in practice**

Our tips   Much of person-centred practice is about having the right attitude. But it is much easier to demonstrate a person-centred approach under exam conditions than it is to do it consistently in everyday practice. The best way to learn this is by getting feedback from patients on how you interact with them in real-life situations.

2.2 Use the general practice consultation to bring about an effective doctor–patient relationship with respect for your patient's autonomy

This means that, as a GP, you should:

2.2.1	**Adopt a patient-centred consultation model that explores the patient's ideas, concerns and expectations, integrates your agenda as a doctor, finds common ground and negotiates a mutual plan for the future**

Our tips   The consultation is central to general practice. One of the most popular and easy-to-use consultation models is Roger Neighbour's five-checkpoint model.[6] In this, five consultation tasks are defined; at each step the GP thinks 'Where shall we make for next and how shall we get there?'

- **Connecting** – establishing a rapport with the patient.

- **Summarising** – using eliciting skills to discover the patient's ideas, concerns, expectations and summarising these back to the patient.

- **Handing over** – agreeing the doctor's and patient's agendas then negotiating, influencing and gift-wrapping these.

- **Safety-netting** – ensuring an appropriate contingency plan has been made.

- **Housekeeping** – clearing away any psychological debris from the consultation to ensure it has no harmful effect on the next.

Continued over

Sharing management decisions with the patient, including potential disagreements over how limited resources should be used, may raise tricky ethical and communication issues, which need to be resolved skilfully without damaging the doctor–patient relationship.

The concept of eliciting the patient's ideas, concerns and expectations at each consultation was first made popular in the mid-1980s by Pendleton and colleagues,[19] and has become an accepted tenet of patient-centred medicine.

See contextual statement 2.01 *The GP Consultation in Practice*, in Chapter 6, for a chart summarising the main consultation models.

2.2.2	**Communicate findings in a comprehensible way, helping patients to reflect on their own concepts and finding common ground for further decision making**
Our tips	Remember there are non-verbal methods of communicating information to patients. These include patient information leaflets (on paper or electronically) and the use of graphs and charts to explain risks and probabilities (e.g. BMI charts or cardiovascular risk charts).

2.2.3	**Make decisions that respect your patient's autonomy**
Our tips	In Western society, patient autonomy has become the overriding ethical principle in most medical decisions, although there are still some notable exceptions to this (e.g. in the areas of child protection and euthanasia).
	In general practice, respecting autonomy involves eliciting and taking into account the patient's ideas, concerns and expectations. It also means involving the patient at all steps of his or her care, including over how uncertainty is managed. Conveying information in a way that is understandable to the patient is key to achieving this – the principle of *informed* consent. A GP should also take steps to maximise the ability of the patient to comprehend the information required to make a decision – the principle of *capacity* to consent.
	Remember that autonomy also applies to the doctor – GPs have the right to refuse to act in a way that they perceive to be against the best interests of their patient, for example.

2.2.4	**Be aware of subjectivity in the medical relationship, from both your patient's side (feelings, values and preferences) and from your own side (self-awareness of values, attitudes and feelings)**
Our tips	Consider keeping a diary of consultations where you and the patient differed over your views on how to proceed. Why did this occur? How did you come to a decision? How could you have handled the situation differently? How did you balance the autonomy of the patient against the needs of the community and your professional duties as a GP?
	Remember you can't please all the people all the time, but you can learn how to handle difficult situations more effectively. You'll inevitably have easier medical relationships with some patients than others. Balint groups explore this area further.[20]

2.3 Communicate, set prioritles and act in partnership

This means that, as a GP, you should:

2.3.1	**Use your skills and attitude to establish a partnership**
Our tips	The first step of the consultation involves establishing a rapport with your patient. It can be helpful to initially focus on an area of common ground that you share with the patient or some personal information you recall (or noted in the records) from a previous encounter; 'How was your visit to see your mother in India, Mrs Patel?'

2.3.2	**Achieve a balance between emotional distance and proximity to your patient**
	Clear professional boundaries exist in the relationship between doctors and patients that must not be crossed (see the GMC's *Good Medical Practice*[2]) although, as with most ethical issues, grey areas exist.
	For example, how would you respond if a patient asks to be your friend on a social media site? Or asks you out for a drink after work? How would your reaction differ if you are working in a remote community where all your social contacts are also your registered patients?

2.4 Provide long-term continuity of care as determined by the needs of your patient, referring to continuing and coordinated care management

This means that, as a GP, you should:

2.4.1	**Understand and master the three aspects of continuity: personal continuity; episodic continuity (making the appropriate medical information available for each patient contact); and continuity of care (24 hours a day and 365 days a year).**
Our tips	Patients have more options than ever before for choosing where they obtain their health care. Most out-of-hours care is provided by organisations outside the practice. In working hours, patients may decide to ring NHS Direct or attend a walk-in centre rather than to visit their GP. Through the 'Choose and Book' system, patients may also choose to be referred to a service outside your locality (e.g. near their place of work).
	Despite these changes, many GPs and patients continue to place great value on the continuity of a personal doctor–patient relationship. Personal continuity is increasingly difficult to provide as the healthcare system becomes more fragmented and complex, so new concepts of continuity are emerging.[21]
	Episodic continuity is affected to a great extent by the effectiveness of the communication between health professionals and their organisations (such as quality of referral processes, correspondence and handovers). One of the goals of the NHS National Programme for IT, which incorporates the centralised electronic patient record, is to use technology to improve episodic continuity.
	Consider ways in which your surgery can optimise these three types of continuity, particularly in challenging situations (e.g. terminal care). Carry out an SEA of a situation where care was compromised by poor continuity. Focus on how it could have been improved.

2.4.2	**Help your patient understand and achieve an appropriate work–life balance**
Our tips	GPs often see patients in whom work-related stress is a contributing factor to their illness. Both physical and mental health can be affected. Also, as the elderly population is rising, greater numbers of workers have additional caring responsibilities at home.[22]
	It is important to remain person centred, however, and recognise that what constitutes an appropriate work–life balance for one individual will not be appropriate for another and that this may change throughout that individual's lifetime.

2.4.3	**Utilise disease registers and data-recording templates effectively for opportunistic and planned monitoring of long-term conditions in order to ensure continuity of care between different healthcare providers**
Our tips	Find out how to record patient data correctly in your practice (the data clerk or the GP in charge of the QOF may be able to help). It is also worth talking to colleagues or visiting other practices to find alternative ways of recording patient data. Review your practice disease registers for a specific chronic disease – how accurate is the register and what are the challenges of ensuring it is both accurate and complete? If you identify a gap in your practice's template collection, why not consider designing one?

Competence 3 – specific problem-solving skills

There are various conceptual models of problem solving in general practice. One of the key early models, developed in this context by Marinker, is the hypothetico-deductive model.[23] This involves the GP formulating a hypothesis to explain the observed symptoms and signs. From the hypothesis a number of predictions of further symptoms and signs are deduced that should be observable as a consequence of the hypothesis.

For example, imagine an otherwise well child presents with a history of right-sided earache and a mild fever for three days. From the history, the GP may formulate the hypothesis that the child is suffering from simple otitis media. The GP will predict that the ear drum will be red and inflamed. This, if confirmed on examination, will confirm the hypothesis and allow the GP to make a further prediction that the child's condition will settle over the next few days. If the child fails to improve as predicted, the original hypothesis must be rejected (a complication may have occurred or the original diagnosis may have been wrong), so the GP informs the parent that if the child does not improve as predicted they should return for another assessment.

3.1 Relate specific decision-making processes to the prevalence and incidence of illness in the community

This means that, as a GP, you should:

3.1.1	Know the prevalence and incidence of disease
Our tips	Prevalence (the proportion of individuals in a population having a disease) and incidence (the number of newly diagnosed cases during a specific time period) differ between primary care, which is a largely unselected population, and secondary care, which has been selected. Disease prevalence and incidence (particularly in terms of possible and probable diagnoses) also differ significantly from one community to another.
	For more information on the common GP conditions described in the curriculum, see Chapter 6, 'The applied knowledge'.

3.1.2   **Know your practice community (age–sex distribution, prevalence of chronic diseases)**

Our tips   How GPs apply their epidemiological knowledge gleaned from a medical textbook to everyday practice will depend on the characteristics of their local community. For example, a GP working in an area with a large student population may expect to see a number of patients presenting with sexual and mental health problems, whereas a GP working in a practice with a predominantly elderly population may expect to see a greater amount of chronic disease.

Knowledge of the community also involves a whole host of other aspects, including genetic, social, psychological, economic, occupational, cultural, religious, educational, language and communication factors.

Established GPs at the practice will have a good idea of the practice community. Carrying out some searches on the practice population or reviewing the QOF chronic disease data can give a good idea of the characteristics of the registered patients.

Find out what specific groups of patients are associated with your practice population (nursing homes, schools, probation hostels, homeless people, drug or substance misusers). Are there any particular issues related to common occupational health issues in your practice area (e.g. mining or industry)?

3.1.3   **Develop your skills in specific decision making (using tools such as clinical reasoning and decision rules)**

Our tips   Start by locating some useful and valid guidelines and decision rules for the more common problems you encounter. For example the Wells criteria,[24] for deep-vein thrombosis (DVT) and pulmonary embolism, and the Ottawa ankle rules,[25] for ankle injury.

Talk to colleagues about the guidelines, decision tools or risk calculators they find easy to apply in practice, but be sure to check their validity to your local population. Some examples:

- cardiovascular risk charts can be found in the back of the BNF

- the British Hypertension Society (www.bhsoc.org) offers downloadable cardiovascular disease (CVD) risk calculators and tables

- the QRisk2 calculator is available at www.qrisk.org

- many practice record systems have built-in decision support software including risk calculators.

3.2 Selectively gather and interpret information from history taking, physical examination and investigations, and apply it to an appropriate management plan in collaboration with your patient

This means that, as a GP, you should:

3.2.1	Know the questions in the history and items in the physical examination that are relevant to the problem presented
Our tips	Unlike a medical student's general clerking, a GP history and examination needs to be focused and accurately target the patient's problem, without being so narrow as to miss potentially important information and signs. Having a disease-based or systems-based approach to history taking and examination does not usually work well in primary care, where patients and their symptoms are unselected. A problem-based approach is generally more effective.[26] This is rather different from the approach adopted in medical school and secondary care, so a transition needs to be made.

3.2.2	Know your patient's relevant context, including family, social and occupational factors
Our tips	Problem solving in general practice is highly context specific. The skills required relate not only to the natural history of the problems themselves, but also to the context in which the problems are encountered, the personal characteristics of the patients and the available resources. Unsurprisingly the best way to find out about a patient's 'relevant context' is to ask the patient. A social history can provide extremely pertinent information; for example, a diagnosis of plantar fasciitis may seem a trivial nuisance to a GP who spends most of the day sitting at his or her desk, but could mean a postman is unable to work for several months.
	It is equally important not to let your knowledge of the patient's family or social background prejudice your decisions and to respect the confidentiality of all the family members and any other patients who may live in the same household.
	Some practice record systems have a handy 'household' function that enables you to pull up the records of other patients registered at the same address.

3.2.3 Know the available investigations and treatment resources

Our tips   This is more than learning about the theory of which tests or treatments you would arrange to investigate a certain condition – it is also about learning the practicalities of how to obtain them.

Find out which investigations and treatments your practice offers patients on site (you may find your practice already has this information handily compiled in a handbook, intranet site or locum folder).

Also, find out where patients need to go to get other investigations or treatments that the practice does not provide – how does this effect how frequently you order them?

3.2.4 Develop your history taking and physical examination skills, and skills in interpreting data

Our tips   Most new GPs will have acquired sound history taking and examination skills during their earlier training. The challenge for trainees is to learn how to adapt these skills to everyday general practice. This is a complex process and involves bringing together a host of clinical skills that may have been learned in different departments over many years. It takes time and practice to get it right. Learning how to consult effectively in the time available (on average about 10 minutes per consultation in most practices) is one of the most challenging aspects of being a GP.

The key investigations used in primary care are listed in Chapter 6, 'The applied knowledge', under the appropriate curriculum statement.

3.2.5 Be willing to involve your patient in the management plan

Our tips   There has been a clear shift over the past few decades away from a traditional paternalistic style of consulting to a more patient-centred style. This learning outcome relates to shared decision making described in the 'Person-centred care' area of competence of the core curriculum statement and is also explored further in contextual statement 2.01 *The GP Consultation in Practice* (see Chapter 6, 'The applied knowledge').

3.3 Adopt appropriate working principles (e.g. incremental investigation, using time as a tool) and tolerate uncertainty

This means that, as a GP, you should:

3.3.1	Adopt skills and attitudes to demonstrate curiosity, diligence and caring
Our tips	The RCGP's motto, *cum scientia caritas* (knowledge with compassion),* illustrates the central importance of care and compassion in high-quality general practice.
	* Others have translated the motto as 'compassion with science' or 'scientific knowledge with caring'.

3.3.2	Adopt stepwise procedures in medical decision making, using time as a diagnostic and therapeutic tool
Our tips	'The art of medicine consists in amusing the patient while nature cures the disease' (Voltaire).
	GPs have the advantage over many hospital-based doctors of being able to establish a personalised relationship with their patients. If a diagnosis is unclear, one option is to allow the passage of time to reveal whether the patient's symptoms and signs develop into a pattern that becomes recognisable as an illness (known as 'using time as a diagnostic tool').
	It is extremely important to consider patient safety when using time as a diagnostic tool – this concept is described as 'safety-netting' in Roger Neighbour's five-checkpoint consultation model.[6] Potentially serious diagnoses must be excluded in order to minimise any risk of harm to the patient from a delay in diagnosis, and the patient should be made aware of the expected natural history of his or her symptoms and any significant variations in the expected pattern that should be reported to a doctor.

3.3.3	Understand and accept the inevitable uncertainty in primary care problem solving and the need for development of strategies that demonstrate this
Our tips	Marinker described GPs as tolerating uncertainty, exploring probability and marginalising danger. Hospital specialists, in contrast, work towards reducing uncertainty, exploring possibility and marginalising error.[23]

A competent GP has the necessary attitudes, knowledge and skills to enable him or her to conduct an effective consultation with a patient, to make an accurate and objective estimation of the risks, and to manage those risks appropriately – 'dealing with uncertainty'. The uncertainty a GP perceives should ideally be proportional to the objective risks that truly exist, although in reality the perception of uncertainty is affected by a number of other factors, including the GP's mental state and previous experiences.

Keeping a reflective diary, to record the consultations where a particularly high degree of uncertainty is felt, will assist you to reflect on the reasons why uncertainty is perceived. Discussing these issues with a mentor or trainer can be a very useful way of identifying some strategies to manage uncertainty and equip you to deal more effectively with the uncertainties that will inevitably arise in the future.

3.4 intervene urgently when necessary

This means that, as a GP, you should:

3.4.1 Develop your skills in specific decision making for emergency situations

Our tips   The adult decision-making process generally involves six stages:

- defining the problem

- collecting information

- exploring the options

- drawing up a plan

- executing the plan

- reviewing the outcome.

In emergency situations, however, decision making is primarily a reactive process and there is insufficient time to go through the stages properly. As a result, it is easy to make bad decisions under pressure.

For this reason, the actions to be taken in an emergency situation should be carefully planned out beforehand so that as few decisions as possible need to be made at the time an emergency event occurs. Practically, this means familiarising yourself with your practice's emergency procedures and plans (e.g. fire, personal attack, flu pandemics) and regularly running through emergency clinical and resuscitation protocols and drills.

3.4.2	**Develop your specific skills for emergency procedures that may occur in primary care situations**

Our tips	Fortunately, emergency procedures are used relatively uncommonly in everyday general practice. For this reason it can be very easy for these skills to get rusty so a strategy for ensuring you remain up to date is important.
	Basic Life Support (BLS) training for adults and children is recommended on a regular basis (at least every 1–2 years), not least because the protocols are frequently updated. If your practice has a defibrillator, you must find out how to use it and check it is properly maintained and serviced. Every practice should have an anaphylaxis kit, particularly when vaccinations are given, and this must also be checked regularly to ensure the drugs and equipment don't go out of date.
	All GP trainees should make arrangements to obtain sufficient out-of-hours experience during their training. The other specific emergency skills will depend on individual practice factors, such as the remoteness of the practice from an emergency department and the characteristics of the local population. Carrying out critical event analyses and team skills assessments will help identify what training the practice team requires.

3.5 Manage conditions that may present early and in an undifferentiated way

This means that, as a GP, you should:

3.5.1	**Know when to wait and reassure, and when to initiate additional diagnostic and therapeutic action**

Our tips	This involves knowing when it is appropriate to wait and see, when to refer, when to arrange a follow-up appointment and when to carry out some investigations to exclude potentially serious diseases. An accurate estimation of risk allows a GP to use his or her feelings of uncertainty to make an appropriate management plan and to successfully share this uncertainty with the patient.
	Be aware of 'red flags'; these are specific symptoms and signs that indicate further action is required. Red flags exist for a range of common symptoms seen in primary care, including back pain, dyspepsia and headache.

3.6 Make effective and efficient use of diagnostic and therapeutic interventions

This means that, as a GP, you should:

3.6.1	**Know that symptoms and signs vary in their predictive value, as do findings from ancillary tests**
Our tips	Predictive value is a fundamental statistical concept. The predictive value of a finding or a test varies with the prevalence (i.e. the pre-test probability) of the disease. This is particularly relevant to primary care where the population has a lower prevalence of serious disease than in secondary care. Generally, the rarer the disease in a population, the lower the positive predictive value of a finding or test.
	This is in contrast with the sensitivity or specificity of a finding or a test, which relates to the test itself and does not depend on the prevalence of the disease.
	Look into the predictive values (both positive and negative) of a few commonly used tests. Examples include D-dimers in suspected DVT, anti-endomysial antibodies in coeliac disease and troponins in the diagnosis of chest pain. How does knowledge of the predictive value of a particular test help with the management of an individual patient?
	The Applied Knowledge Test (AKT) component of the MRCGP tests knowledge of basic statistics. Candidates should learn the definitions and concepts of the common terms used in evidence-based health care – see Chapter 6, 'The applied knowledge', for useful resources.

3.6.2	**Understand the cost-efficiency and cost–benefit of tests and treatments**
Our tips	In health care, cost-efficiency is a measure of the total spending for a service (or group of services associated with a specific patient population) compared against a clinical outcome over a specified time period. A cost–benefit analysis is used for determining which alternative intervention is likely to provide the greatest health improvement for a proposed amount of investment.

Competence 4 – a comprehensive approach

An effective GP must be able to manage the multiple complaints and co-morbidities of his or her patients. When a patient seeks medical advice, he or she has become ill as a person and may not be able to differentiate between the effects of his or her various conditions. The challenge of addressing multiple health issues simultaneously requires GPs to develop the skills needed to both interpret the issues and to prioritise them in partnership with the patient. GPs also provide rehabilitation for their patients and, in the end phase of a patient's life, palliative care. A GP must be able to coordinate the care provided by other healthcare professionals and agencies.

4.1 Manage multiple complaints and pathologies simultaneously, for both acute and chronic health problems

This means that, as a GP, you should:

4.1.1	Understand the concept of co-morbidity in a patient
Our tips	Co-morbidity describes the effect of any other diseases of an individual patient other than the disease primarily being considered. It is particularly relevant in the care of the elderly and also increasingly a matter of concern in patients suffering from mental health problems, who often have neglected physical health problems.

4.1.2	Develop your skills to manage the concurrent health problems experienced by your patient through identification, exploration, negotiation, acceptance and prioritisation
Our tips	Keep a record of a handful of patients you see with four or more active problems – then review their notes and medications, and consider how these problems may interact, both physically and in psychosocial ways.

4.1.3	Develop your skills in using the medical record and other information
Our tips	Early on in your training have a tutorial on how to use your practice computer system. Ask colleagues to review your entries and provide feedback on ways you might improve them.

4.1.4	**Develop your skills and attitudes so that you seek and use the best evidence in practice**

Our tips	In this outcome, the *attitude* is about wanting to practise evidence-based health care on a regular basis.
	The two main aspects to this *skill* are being able to interpret the evidence, so as to have an answer to your question, and then being able to apply it in practice. This involves knowing where to look and learning how to ask the right question. Good publications in which to find high-quality evidence include the Cochrane Library, Clinical Evidence, Best Evidence and in peer-reviewed journals. (Two journals particularly relevant to general practice are the *British Journal of General Practice* and the *British Medical Journal*.)
	The RCGP hosts an e-learning package for GP trainees on evidence-based health care at www.e-GP.org. Other useful resources include the Centre for Evidence Based Medicine (www.cebm.net), which has resources for developing evidence-based healthcare skills. NHS Evidence (www.evidence.nhs.uk) hosts many evidence-based articles and guidelines.

4.2 Promote health and wellbeing by applying health promotion and disease prevention strategies appropriately

This means that, as a GP, you should:

4.2.1	**Understand the concept of health**

Our tips	The World Health Organization defines health as 'a state of complete physical, mental and social well-being and not merely the absence of disease or infirmity'.[27] This definition highlights how health should be considered holistically, rather than just focusing on physical health.

4.2.2	**Know how to promote health on an individual basis as part of the consultation**

Our tips	There are numerous health promotion opportunities in a consultation. A few common examples include smoking cessation, diet and exercise advice, sexual health screening, and cancer screening.

Continued over

All of the above examples require patients to change their lifestyles. The real skill comes in tailoring the messages to the individual patient and framing them in a way the patient will be willing and able to assimilate and act on. This requires a degree of experience (i.e. practice!) and the ability to manage the barriers that often prevent doctors from addressing lifestyle factors – such as shortage of time and the belief (which is generally false) that raising these issues might adversely affect the doctor–patient relationship. In reality, patients expect their doctors to talk to them about their lifestyles and there is substantial evidence to support the effectiveness of these interventions.

4.2.3	**Know how to promote health through a health promotion or disease prevention programme within the primary care setting**
Our tips	As well as promoting health in the consultation, GPs and their teams promote health in their own practices.
	There are a number of established disease prevention programmes already in operation in the UK. These include vaccination programmes and screening programmes for cervical cancer, breast cancer and bowel cancer. Some of these take place in practices and others are managed by other organisations. Advice from GPs is often very influential in patients' decisions about whether to engage with these programmes.

4.2.4	**Understand the role of the GP in health promotion activities in the community**
Our tips	GPs have a responsibility to improve health in their local communities, often working with other organisations (e.g. clinical commissioning groups, local authorities and organisations from the third sector).
	The ultimate aim of a public health initiative is to improve the health and wellbeing of the *whole* population; reducing health inequality is an essential part of this.
	This outcome is explored further in Chapter 6, 'The applied knowledge' – see clinical example 3.01 *Healthy People: promoting health and preventing disease*.

4.2.5	**Understand and recognise the importance of ethical tensions between the needs of the individual and the community, and act appropriately**
Our tips	Keep a log of any resource dilemmas that arise in your practice, and discuss them with your trainer or learning group. What are the basic ethical principles involved and how can you address the dilemma?
	Consider the concept of 'opportunity cost' in health care – this is the cost paid, both economically and in terms of people's wellbeing, when we give up something in order to get something else.

4.3 Manage and coordinate health promotion, prevention, cure, care, rehabilitation and palliation

This means that, as a GP, you should:

4.3.1	**Understand the complex nature of health problems in general practice**
Our tips	Consider how complexity in general practice exists at various levels. First, the evidence base that underpins medicine is ever expanding, making it increasingly difficult for generalists to keep a broad overview across the breadth of general practice. Second, patients are presenting with more complex health problems, both in terms of the numbers of problems each individual may develop over time and their more sophisticated expectations of investigation and treatment. Third, the professional role of the GP is also becoming more complex. GPs are now expected to not only provide cost-effective care for the patients in front of them, whatever they may present with, but also to take responsibility for the organisation of their practice and the successful running of their team. Beyond this, GPs must consider the wider needs of the population in which they work and actively contribute to innovation and quality improvement in the healthcare system.

4.3.2	**Understand the variety of possible approaches**
Our tips	No two patients are the same, so a successful GP needs a repertoire of skills and to be able to select which to use with each particular patient. Patients can be young, old, well, ill, poorly informed or well informed about their health, anxious or laidback. People come from a range of different cultures and nationalities, and hold very different views on the determinants of ill health. All of these factors contribute to each patient's individual complexity.

Continued over

There are also inter-professional variations. Try sitting in with different healthcare professionals to observe some of this variety. You will notice that some colleagues seem particularly adept at communicating with particular types of patients about their health. If there are only a few other professionals at your practice, consider arranging a swap with a colleague at another practice to broaden your experience.

4.3.3   **Use different approaches for an individual patient and modify these according to an individual's need**

Our tips   In addition to a portfolio of skills used during the conventional office-based consultations, think about skills needed for alternative types of consultation (e.g. drop-in services, home visits, telephone or email consultations, internet-based advice, blogs, etc.).

4.3.4   **Be able to coordinate teamwork in primary care**

Our tips   There is lots of theory written about teamwork. Relevant models for general practice include:

- Myers–Briggs personality profiles [28]

- Belbin's team roles [8, 29]

- Bruce Tuckman's group development model [30]

- Maslow's motivational needs hierarchy model [31]

- leadership styles.

The website www.businessballs.com contains information on these models of team theory and leadership, and offers some games and exercises to encourage team building. A GP's role includes coordinating and leading a team – observe and evaluate others doing it and talk to your trainer or practice manager about creating opportunities for you to try out being a team leader on a practice project. Remember to ask for and record constructive feedback.

Competence 5 – community orientation

GPs, as family and community doctors, have a responsibility that stretches beyond the boundaries of a consultation with an individual patient. The work of a GP is determined by the make-up of his or her community and therefore GPs must understand the characteristics of the community in which they work, including socio-economic and health features. Healthcare systems are rationed in some form in all societies, and GPs have a clinical, ethical and moral duty to influence health policy in their community.

5.1 Reconcile the health needs of individual patients and the health needs of the community in which they live, balancing these with available resources

This means that, as a GP, you should:

5.1.1	Understand the health needs of communities through the epidemiological characteristics of their populations
Our tips	To provide effective services, the local GPs, the practices and the local NHS must tailor their services to the particular needs of their communities (see outcome 3.1.2 in this chapter). This requires the ability to understand and interpret local health data, including health outcomes and feedback from the public on their experience of using services.

5.1.2	Understand the interrelationships between health and social care
Our tips	In the past, the various agencies involved in health and social care have not succeeded in coordinating their responses to patient needs. This has led to people being assessed repeatedly and valuable information being lost. People often complain that they are not kept informed about what is happening with their health care.
	Find out about the Single Assessment Process (SAP) that was introduced following the publication of the National Service Framework for Older People.[32] A key principle is that there is a single person-centred and holistic assessment to which the various health and social services contribute.

| 5.1.3 | **Understand the impact of poverty, ethnicity and local epidemiology on a local community's health** |

Our tips   The health of people in the UK has dramatically improved over the past two centuries. In 1841, average life expectancy was 40.2 years for men and 42.2 for women – but by 2000 it had almost doubled to 75.6 and 80.3 years respectively.[33]

Despite these huge overall improvements, there are remarkable differences in the health of different groups and the higher an individual's social status, the longer he or she is likely to live. For example, a girl born in Kensington and Chelsea has a life expectancy of 87.8 years, more than ten years higher than a girl born in Glasgow City whose life expectancy is 77.1 years.[34] There are also significant differences in other health statuses relating to ethnicity and other socioeconomic factors, such as education and unemployment.

| 5.1.4 | **Be aware of inequalities in healthcare provision** |

Our tips   Forty years ago a GP called Julian Tudor Hart proposed 'the inverse care law'.[35] This describes how socioeconomically deprived people, who need health care the most, are the least likely to get it. In contrast, those with less need for health care tend to use the health services more effectively.

Familiarise yourself with the specific healthcare issues and inequalities affecting the homeless, asylum seekers and refugees.

The King's Fund provides reports on the impact of inequalities in healthcare provision (www.kingsfund.org.uk). Regrettably, 'postcode lotteries' still exist in health care.

| 5.1.5 | **Understand the structure of the healthcare system and its economic limitations** |

Our tips   You are doing well if you are able to gain a full understanding of the structure of the NHS! This is because it is a large and complex organisation, is subject to change and varies considerably across the four home nations of the UK.

There are regional NHS websites that provide useful summaries of the structure of the NHS:

- England – www.nhs.uk/NHSEngland/thenhs
- Scotland – www.show.scot.nhs.uk

- Wales – www.wales.nhs.uk

- Northern Ireland – www.hscni.net.

5.1.6	**Understand the roles of the other professionals involved in community policy relating to health**

Our tips
To develop integrated services and to address the social determinants of ill health, GPs need to work with colleagues from a range of clinical and non-clinical backgrounds, including public health organisations, social services, local authorities and third-sector organisations.[36] To be effective, GPs must appreciate the contributions of these colleagues to local healthcare services and the factors that result in effective joint-working.[37]

National clinical organisations of relevance to population health include:

- the Faculty of Public Health of the Royal College of Physicians (www.fphm. org.uk), which is the standard-setting body for specialists in public health

- the Health Protection Agency (www.hpa.org.uk), which is an independent body that protects the health and wellbeing of the population. At the time of writing, there is a possibility that its functions may be transferred to other bodies as part of NHS reorganisation

- the National Institute for Health and Clinical Excellence (www.nice.org. uk), which is an independent organisation responsible for providing national guidance on the promotion of good health and the prevention and treatment of ill health in England and Wales. This process includes appraising treatments for cost-effectiveness and recommending treatments for the NHS.

Following devolution and the Health and Social Care Bill (2012), significant differences now exist in the organisation of public health in the four UK home nations – find out the arrangements in your region.

5.1.7	**Contribute to service management and service improvement in your local health community, as well as in your own practice**

Our tips
As well as improving their own practices, GPs are taking on an increasing role in re-designing and improving local NHS services to meet healthcare priorities, particularly in England where GPs are taking on formal commissioning responsibilities. To perform this role successfully, GPs require a solid understanding of local health data, patient safety, quality improvement, efficiency and patient feedback.

Continued over

If you work in England, consider contacting your local commissioning group for more information on how to get involved.

For further information on this outcome, see Chapter 6, clinical example 3.01 *Healthy People: promoting health and preventing disease.*

5.1.8	**Understand the importance of practice- and community-based information in the quality assurance of your individual practice**
Our tips	Regular audit and evaluation of your own performance are central parts of continuing professional development. As part of your five-yearly revalidation as a GP, you will be required to present data relating to the quality of your work. On an individual level, this includes significant event and other audit data, prescribing and referrals data, patient satisfaction survey data, and 360° feedback from colleagues.
	On a practice level, the QOF seeks to raise standards of care by rewarding practices financially for hitting targets set either by central government or locally. It incentivises practices to collect and review practice-level data on a number of common long-term conditions, (e.g. asthma, diabetes, epilepsy, hypertension, hypothyroidism, depression, dementia, etc.). QOF results for individual practices can be viewed at: www.qof.ic.nhs.uk.

5.1.9	**Understand how the healthcare system can be used by the patient and the doctor (referral procedures, co-payments, sick leave, legal issues, etc.) in their own context**
Our tips	People do not only use the healthcare system to obtain health care. Many people visit their GP with a different agenda. Here are some of the more common non-medical agendas:

- to obtain a sickness certificate

- to get their passport application signed

- to request a letter or medical report

- to attend for a medical examination (e.g. for life insurance).

Arrange a tutorial on the sickness certification system ('fit notes') and common medical reports that are required for those claiming benefits.

5.1.10   **Reconcile the needs of your individual patients with the needs of the community in which they live**

Our tips   Part of the traditional GP role in the NHS is that of 'gatekeeper'. The idea of GPs rationing access to health care is politically sensitive in the era of patient choice. In recent years, there have been attempts to formalise this 'rationing' task within Primary Care Organisations, through the use of referral management centres and 'low-priority treatment' statements. Despite this, making effective use of NHS resources remains an implicit part of a modern GP's role and will be a greater responsibility for GPs in England under clinically led commissioning. However, the emphasis has increasingly shifted towards that of 'navigator' – guiding the patient through the health service in the most effective and safe way possible.

A key aspect of the community-oriented nature of general practice is the role that GPs play in the rationing of healthcare resources and the influencing of health policy in the community; the NHS has finite resources and a significant proportion of NHS spending happens in primary care. GPs need to be able to balance the needs of individual patients against the needs of the whole community they serve.

5.1.11   **Understand your role as a GP in the commissioning of health care**

Our tips   In **England**, GPs are being given formal responsibility for commissioning health care – that is, the process of assessing the needs of a population, planning and procuring services for that population, and then monitoring and evaluating the impact of those services. GPs will carry out this role by working with other professionals and the public in their local commissioning groups.

Health is a devolved power, however, and clinically led commissioning is currently only being introduced in England. In Scotland, Wales and Northern Ireland, GPs have not yet been given formal responsibility for commissioning. However, GPs in these nations have traditionally been more closely involved in the management of local services than in England.

In **Scotland**, there are 14 health boards with responsibility for commissioning and monitoring the performance of NHS trusts. The Scottish government has indicated that it might give GPs more commissioning powers.

In **Wales**, seven health boards have responsibility for commissioning, and there is separation between commissioning and provision of health care.

In **Northern Ireland**, there is an integrated health and social care system. This consists of four boards that commission and monitor services.

Continued over

Whatever the regional arrangements, integrated services cannot be commissioned effectively without the full participation of all the healthcare professionals involved and the public. This requires GPs to engage with others in local GP practices, community teams, specialist teams and hospitals to evaluate data on patient experience and outcomes, to identify potential improvements and to design improved systems of care.

Competence 6 – a holistic approach

Holism in general practice involves the integration of the physical, psychological and social components of health problems and is well established as being central to good consulting practice.

6.1 Use biopsychosocial models and take into account cultural and existential dimensions

This means that, as a GP, you should:

6.1.1	Know the holistic concept and implications for your patients' care
Our tips	Kemper defines holism as 'caring for the whole person in the context of the person's values, their family beliefs, their family system and their culture in the larger community, and considering a range of therapies based on the evidence of their benefits and cost'.[38] It can also be described as the integration of physical, psychological and social components of health problems in making diagnoses and planning management.
	The concept of holism and the key references are summarised very well in the full text of the core curriculum statement 1.0 *Being a General Practitioner.*

6.1.2	Understand your patient as a biopsychosocial 'whole'
Our tips	The RCGP's triaxial model (biological, psychological and social) forms a basic framework for a GP to consider a patient holistically, including physical, emotional, family, social and environmental circumstances.[39] Cultural and existential issues (those relating to people's experience of existence) are also considered part of holism but are not explicitly covered by the triaxial model.
	Of course, describing patients in this abstract way risks reducing them to theoretical concepts – when all is said and done, patients, like their doctors, are people first!

6.1.3	**Develop the skills to transform holistic understanding into practical measures**
Our tips	This competency requires appropriate knowledge of ethnic and cultural behaviour including specific practical knowledge (e.g. nutrition, naming systems, religion, attitudes toward illness, death, and pregnancy). If you work in a community with a low level of cultural diversity, this does not mean you won't need to devote as much effort to learning about various cultural groups – in fact you will have to try harder to acquire this knowledge as your experience of meeting such patients will be more limited than GPs in more diverse communities.

6.1.4	**Know the cultural background and beliefs of your patient, in so far as they are relevant to health care**
Our tips	This is partly about having an awareness of the cultural aspects relevant to particular groups of patients you may see, and partly about gaining specific knowledge of *individual* patient's beliefs. For example, you may be at a loss to explain why a patient seems reluctant to take the lansoprazole capsules you have prescribed for their heartburn, until you discover the capsules contain gelatine, which the patient is unwilling to consume for religious reasons.
	Few people are reluctant to discuss their culture or beliefs yet many GPs worry excessively about causing offence if they ask about them – we would suggest it is far better to plead ignorance and ask your patient, rather than make assumptions!

6.1.5	**Show tolerance and understanding of your patients' experiences, beliefs, values and expectations as they affect healthcare delivery**
Our tips	Identify a specific situation in which you have struggled with being tolerant and understanding towards a patient. This can be a sensitive subject, so you may prefer to reflect on this alone, or preferably discuss it with a trainer or trusted colleague – try to identify what happened, then why the difficulties arose, and come up with some alternative ways of dealing with the situation.

The three essential features

The essential application features are about *you*, the doctor. They are important factors that are always present in the background of a consultation and exert a strong effect on how a GP's knowledge and skills are applied in everyday general practice.

1 Contextual features

These features include the environment in which a doctor practices, the working conditions, the community, local culture, financial and regulatory frameworks and guidelines; the impact of workload and the practice facilities; the particular context of the individual patient and his or her family and background.

2 Attitudinal features

These features include the doctor's own attitudes and capabilities; the ability to identify ethical aspects of clinical practice and to understand his or her personal ethics and values; achieving a good balance between work and private life.

3 Scientific features

These features include the doctor adopting a critical and evidence-based approach to daily practice and maintaining this through continuing learning, professional development and quality improvement.

Essential feature 1 – contextual features

Every GP needs to understand how his or her own working context, as a doctor, may influence the quality of the care he or she provides.

This requires an understanding of the context of general practice and the environment in which GPs work, including the local working conditions, community, culture, financial and regulatory frameworks and guidelines; the impact of workload and the practice facilities; the particular context of the individual patient and his or her family and background.

EF 1.1	**Understanding the impact of the local community (including socioeconomic and workplace factors, geography and culture) on your patient care**
Our tips	Reflect on the features of your practice's local community that particularly influence the delivery of patient care – how does the community exert this influence and are there any factors that you can modify? Consider how this contrasts with other practices; practices may be located in inner-city or rural communities, in affluent or deprived areas, and so on. Remember that 'no man is an island'.*

* John Donne (1572–1631).

EF 1.2	**Awareness of the impact of overall workload on the care given to the individual patient and the facilities (e.g. staff, equipment) available to deliver that care**
Our tips	What length appointments does your practice offer patients and why? Do all the GPs offer the same-length consultations? Review the evidence that longer consultation times provide improved quality of care.[40] Consider the factors that stretch your practice's ability to deliver care (demand for appointments, staff holidays, requests for urgent home visits, unexpected sick leave, etc.) and the plans in place to address these, as well as the practice-based factors that link to high-quality care.

EF 1.3	**Understanding the financial, regulatory and legal frameworks in which you provide health care at a practice level**
Our tips	This includes being familiar with relevant aspects of common law, employment law, important acts of parliament and professional guidelines for best practice. It also involves gaining an understanding of how general practices are financed and the various types of GP contract. Speak to the senior partner or the practice manager about how these various frameworks are implemented and managed in your practice.

EF 1.4   **Understanding the impact of your personal, home and working environment on the care that you provide**

Our tips   Consider how the fabric of the building you work in affects the care you offer patients. This includes the number of available consulting and treatment rooms, the size and comfort of the waiting rooms (e.g. do you have easily accessible chairs for infirm patients?), access for those with disability, and the equipment you have in the practice (e.g. is there an ECG machine and a spirometer or do you have to persuade patients to attend the local hospital or diagnostic centre for these investigations?). It is almost inevitable that, at some point in your career, factors in your home life will have an impact on your professional life.

Essential Feature 2 – attitudinal features

Every GP needs to understand his or her professional capabilities, feelings and ethics, and the impact these may have on patient care.

This understanding requires the GP to be aware of his or her own attitudes and capabilities; the ability to identify ethical aspects of clinical practice and to understand his or her personal ethics and values; and achieving a good balance between work and private life.

EF 2.1	**Awareness of your own capabilities and values**
Our tips	Reflective practice is an essential skill in modern professional practice, and a significant aspect of this involves gaining an understanding of your own values. You can also assess your capabilities objectively (e.g. through the use of rating scales and assessments) and from feedback from others.
	The Johari window,[41,*] is a useful conceptual tool for assessing and improving your self-awareness. You can find it on the Businessballs website (www.businessballs.com).
	* Interestingly, Luft and Ingham created the name 'Johari' in the 1960s by combining their first names, Joe and Harry.

EF 2.2	**Being able to identify the ethical aspects of your clinical practice (prevention, diagnostics, therapy, factors that influence lifestyles)**
Our tips	The four ethical principles of autonomy, beneficence, non-maleficence and justice are a good foundation for making ethical judgements. Be alert to the classic ethical dilemmas of general practice – areas such as abortion, use of chaperones, confidentiality, euthanasia, genetic testing, informed consent, rationing of health care and whistle-blowing are fairly obvious arenas for ethical debates in the Clinical Skills Assessment (CSA) and for case-based discussion (CbD). A learning group is an ideal forum for discussing cases that raise complex ethical issues as it encourages members to form their own opinions and exposes people to alternative ideas and perspectives.
	Less obvious ethical issues crop up all the time in day-to-day practice. For example, considering to what extent to twist a patient's arm when attempting to persuade him or her to stop engaging in what you believe to be a harmful activity, such as smoking, involves a judgement based on the conflicting principles of autonomy and beneficence.
	Familiarise yourself with the professional ethical guidelines and legal frameworks within which healthcare decisions should be made, such as the GMC's document *Good Medical Practice*,[2] the Equality Act 2010, the Mental Capacity Act 2005 and the Mental Health Act 1983.

EF 2.3	**Awareness of self: understanding that your own attitudes and feelings are important determinants of how you practice**

Our tips

'*Know yourself*' was inscribed at the entrance to the Temple of Apollo at Delphi – Apollo was considered to be an ancient god of healing.

A reflective diary can help to identify situations in which your attitudes and feelings influenced your practice. This should include both positive and negative experiences.

Psychological concepts such as transference (the patient unconsciously transferring feelings arising from another relationship to the GP) and counter-transference (the GP experiencing feelings through identification with the emotions, experiences or problems of the patient) can provide some useful insights. Consider how these phenomena may affect your consultations (especially if a patient makes you feel particularly angry, upset or anxious but you aren't sure why).

EF 2.4	**Valuing and encouraging the contribution of others**

Our tips

This includes not only listening to, valuing and reflecting on the contributions of other GPs, but also the contributions of patients, professional colleagues and all the other people with whom you have a working relationship.

It also involves an appreciation of multidisciplinary working (i.e. adopting a shared leadership approach and recognising the limitations of your own abilities) in order to deliver the best care for patients. More broadly, it includes the attitudes you need to engage successfully with patients and the public in improving the organisation of the practice and in re-designing and commissioning local services.

EF 2.5	**Being prepared to participate in service management and improvement**

Our tips

It is important that every GP is prepared to participate in improving services for patients for several reasons:

- it ensures all the clinicians are engaged with the process of change – this is important when it comes to persuading individuals to change their practice. Without this engagement, the attempt to implement change is likely to fail

- it ensures that the widest possible range of clinical experience has been captured in the decision-making process; every team member brings their own piece of the jigsaw, to reveal the bigger picture

Continued over

- it broadens and deepens the pool of resources and skills available to the team

- it encourages innovation and encourages novel suggestions for providing a more effective, high-quality service.

This duty to participate in service improvement applies regardless of whether you are a salaried GP, a locum, a partner or an out-of-hours GP.

EF 2.6	**Justifying and clarifying personal ethics**
Our tips	Spend some time thrashing out your thoughts on some of the common ethical issues that are bound to come up as a working GP. Then, when you meet these situations, you will have an opportunity to reflect and further develop your personal ethics. If you don't take time to reflect on your actions when ethical issues arise in practice, you may not be aware if your behaviour starts to deviate from the values you support.
	Review your practice's policies on accepting gifts from patients and for ensuring financial probity within the practice.

EF 2.7	**Being aware of the interaction between work and your private life; striving for a good balance between them**
Our tips	Work–life balance is important for GPs as well as their patients. A good balance will depend on your personal circumstances and personality although every GP should be aware of the phenomenon of 'burnout' and ways to prevent it. Burnout is a syndrome of emotional exhaustion, depersonalisation, low productivity and low achievement. It is a particular problem in the medical profession.[42]
	All GPs, like their patients, become ill at some point in their careers. But many GPs avoid consulting their own GP and may have inappropriate 'corridor consultations' with colleagues instead. They often find backdoor ways to obtain health care and are at risk of self-diagnosing, self-prescribing and self-referring. Poor doctor health not only affects the individual concerned; it also adversely affects the care of patients, increases healthcare costs, and makes the lives of colleagues, family and friends more difficult.
	The RCGP's Health for Health Professionals online courses explore these issues and highlight sources of support for medics who are ill and for the doctors who look after them (www.elearning.rcgp.org.uk).

Essential Feature 3 – scientific features

Every GP should adopt a critical and evidence-based approach to his or her work, maintaining this through lifelong learning and a commitment to quality improvement.

This requires the adoption of a critical and evidence-based approach to daily practice, maintaining this through continuing learning, professional development and quality improvement.

EF 3.1	**Familiarity with the general principles, methods and concepts of scientific research and the fundamentals of statistics (incidence, prevalence, predicted value, etc.)**
Our tips	The RCGP's motto, *cum scientia caritas* (knowledge with compassion), illustrates that high-quality general practice requires care and compassion applied with a rational, scientific, evidence-based approach.
	The RCGP's Evidence-Based Practice course in the e-GP resource introduces the basic statistics that GPs needs to know and shows how this know-how can be applied to everyday primary care scenarios (available at www.e-GP.org).

EF 3.2	**Knowing the scientific backgrounds of pathology, symptoms and diagnosis, therapy and prognosis, epidemiology, decision theory, theories about the forming of hypotheses and problem solving, and preventive health care**
Our tips	This is clearly a huge area and most of the detailed knowledge is covered in Chapter 6, 'The applied knowledge'. However, you may need to look outside the curriculum to find the scientific and theoretical background to decision theory, hypothesis forming and problem solving.

EF 3.3	**Reading and assessing medical literature critically and putting the lessons from the literature into practice**
Our tips	There are several good resources, including websites and books, on critical appraisal. Look at the RCGP curriculum resources website for some of these: www.rcgp.org.uk/curriculum.
	Also consider:

- does your practice have a journal club?

- if so, how do you identify which papers to read?

Continued over

- do you know how to find high-quality papers that answer your (well-framed) clinical questions? Look at: www.cebm.net

- some adopt a 'scan the key journals' approach, whereas others focus on articles based on clinical interest (what are the benefits and risks of these approaches?)

- try out the 'journal watch' services offered by some publications and websites such as the RCGP (www.rcgp.org.uk)

- the RCGP Essential Knowledge Updates programme provides six-monthly online updates on new and changing knowledge in general practice (www.elearning.rcgp.org.uk)

- classroom-based updating courses are a popular way to keep your awareness of recent developments up to date, although you are relying on other people to set the agenda.

EF 3.4	**Developing and maintaining continuing learning and quality improvement**
Our tips	Trainee GPs must demonstrate ongoing learning through regular reviews of the evidence in their Trainee ePortfolio (https://eportfolio.rcgp.org.uk). For more information on this, see Chapter 4, 'Succeeding at the MRCGP'.
	All NHS GPs are now required to undergo annual appraisal and five-yearly revalidation. Revalidation requires all GPs to maintain an e-portfolio, including evidence of learning activity, performance and a Personal Development Plan.
	The RCGP Revalidation ePortfolio (https://gpeportfolio.rcgp.org.uk) has been developed for qualified GPs. This facilitates the process of gathering evidence, recording CPD credits, and guides the doctor through the appraisal and revalidation processes.
	Quality improvement involves not only personal development but also improving the service offered by the whole practice and the local community. Find out if your practice has an up-to-date practice development plan and look at the RCGP website (www.rcgp.org.uk) for more information on quality improvement.

Using the areas of competence to plan learning

An example using the areas of competence to plan learning activities on cancer and palliative care is included in Table 5.1.

Table 5.1

Using the curriculum domains to plan learning

Example learning activities relating to curriculum statement 3.09 *End-of-Life Care*

Area of competence	Essential application features		
	Contextual	Attitudinal	Scientific
1 Primary care management	Read the *Gold Standards Framework for Palliative Care*[43] documents	Discussion with trainer on how my personal experience affects my management	Read textbook section on how to prescribe opioids and other palliative medications
2 Person-centred approach	Find out how to inform the out-of-hours service about a palliative patient	Read up on the issues around Advanced Directives and capacity to consent	Tutorial arranged on models for the doctor–patient relationship
3 Specific problem-solving skills	Arrange role-plays with actors or colleagues on day release to practise breaking bad news	Discussion planned in Learning Group on the ethics around end-of-life and euthanasia	Go over how to set up a syringe driver with the district nurse
4 A comprehensive approach	Read up on benefits available for the terminally ill (and the DS1500 form)	Journal club discussion on qualitative research into patients' views on loss of dignity and dying	Review textbook section on the causes of reduced pain threshold (e.g. anxiety, constipation)
5 Community orientation	Arrange a day with the Macmillan nurse, visiting patients dying at home	Reflect on the NHS end-of-life care strategy	Identify local risk factors for cancer and prevalence from practice QOF data
6 A holistic approach	Organise a case-based discussion with trainer on the needs of carers in the practice	Ask colleagues how they would ask a palliative patient about spiritual care needs	Read up on the key models of bereavement and important sources of support

References

1   *The European Definition of General Practice/Family Medicine*. Barcelona: WONCA Europe, 2002.

2   General Medical Council. *Good Medical Practice*. London: GMC, 2006, updated 2009, www.gmc-uk.org [accessed May 2012].

3   Royal College of General Practitioners, General Practitioners Committee. *Good Medical Practice for General Practitioners*. London: RCGP, 2008, www.rcgp.org.uk/pdf/PDS_Good_Medical_Practice_for_GPs_July_2008.pdf [accessed May 2012].

4   Eve R. Meeting educational needs in general practice: learning with PUNs and DENs. *Education for General Practice* 2000; **11**: 73–9.

5   Luft J, Ingham H. The Johari window, a graphic model of interpersonal awareness. In: *Proceedings of the Western Training Laboratory in Group Development*. Los Angeles: UCLA, 1955.

6   Neighbour R. *The Inner Consultation*. Lancaster: MTP Press, 1987.

7   Wilson V, Pirrie A. *Multidisciplinary Teamworking. Beyond the barriers? A review of the issues*. SCRE Research Report No 96, 2000, https://dspace.gla.ac.uk/bitstream/1905/227/1/096.pdf [accessed May 2012].

8   Belbin R M. *Management Teams: why they succeed or fail*. Oxford: Butterworth-Heinemann, 1981.

9   Primary Care Commissioning, www.pcc.nhs.uk [accessed May 2012].

10 Campbell H, Hotchkiss R, Bradshaw N, *et al*. Integrated care pathways. *British Medical Journal* 1998; **316(7125)**: 133–7.

11 RCGP curriculum statement 3.2: *Patient Safety*. London: RCGP, 2006.

12 Rees Jones I, Doyle L, Berney L, *et al*. *Decision-Making in Primary Care: patients as partners in resource allocation*. London: St George's Medical School, 2003.

13 Stewart M (ed.). *Patient-Centered Medicine: transforming the clinical method*. Thousand Oaks, CA: Sage, 1995.

14 Kinnersley P, Stott N, Peters T J, *et al*. The patient-centredness of consultations and outcome in primary care. *British Journal of General Practice* 1999; **49(446)**: 711–16.

15 Greenhalgh T, Hurwitz B (eds). *Narrative Based Medicine*. London: BMJ Books, 1998.

16 Helman C G. Disease versus illness in general practice. *Journal of the Royal College of General Practitioners* 1981; **31**: 548–62.

17 Rosenstock I. *Historical Origins of the Health Belief Model*. Health Education Monographs Vol. 2, No. 4, 1974.

18 Tamm M E. Models of health and disease. *British Journal of Medical Psychology* 1993; **66**: 213–28.

19 Pendleton D, Schofield T, Tate P, *et al*. *The Consultation: an approach to learning and teaching*. Oxford: Oxford University Press, 1984.

20   Balint M. *The Doctor, His Patient and the Illness*. London: Pitman Medical Publishing, 1964.

21   Freeman G, Hjortdahl P. What future for continuity of care in general practice? *British Medical Journal* 1997; **314**: 1870–3.

22   www.unison.org.uk [accessed May 2012].

23   Marinker M, Peckham M (eds). *Clinical Futures*. London: BMJ Books, 1998.

24   Wells P S, Anderson D R, Rodger M, *et al.* Derivation of a simple clinical model to categorize patients' probability of pulmonary embolism: increasing the model's utility with the SimpliRED D-dimer. *Journal of Thrombosis and Haemostasis* 2000; **83(3)**: 416–20.

25   Dowling S, Spooner C H, Liang Y, *et al.* Accuracy of Ottawa ankle rules to exclude fractures of the ankle and midfoot in children: a meta-analysis. *Academic Emergency Medicine* 2009; **16(4)**: 277–87.

26   Deighan M. *RCGP Curriculum for General Practice: learning and teaching guide*. London: RCGP, 2006.

27   *Constitution of the World Health Organization*. Geneva: WHO, 1946.

28   Briggs Myers I. *Manual: The Myers–Briggs Type Indicator*. Palo Alto, CA: CPP, 1962.

29   www.belbin.com [accessed May 2012].

30   Tuckman B W. Developmental sequence in small groups. *Psychology Bulletin* 1965; **63**: 384–99.

31   Maslow A. *Motivation and Personality*. New York: Harper, 1970.

32   Department of Health. *National Service Framework for Older People*. London: DH, 2001, www.dh.gov.uk [accessed May 2012].

33   House of Commons Health Committee, Third Report of Session 2008–09, Health Inequalities Volume I, www.publications.parliament.uk/pa/cm200809/cmselect/cmhealth/286/286.pdf [accessed May 2012].

34   Office of National Statistics. Life Expectancy by Local Authority, 1992–2006, www.statistics.gov.uk/hub/index.html [accessed May 2012].

35   Tudor Hart J. The inverse care law. *Lancet* 1971; **i**: 405–12.

36   The King's Fund. *Tackling Inequalities in General Practice*. London: King's Fund, 2010, www.kingsfund.org.uk/current_projects/gp_inquiry/dimensions_of_care/inequalities.html [accessed May 2012].

37   Cameron A, Lart R. Factors promoting and obstacles hindering joint working: a systematic review of the research evidence. *Journal of Integrated Care* 2003; **11(2)**: 9–17.

38   Kemper K J. Holistic pediatrics = good medicine. *Pediatrics* 2000; **105**: 214–18.

39   Working Party of the Royal College of General Practitioners. *The Triaxial Model of the Consultation*. London: RCGP, 1972.

40   Silverman J, Kinnersley P. Calling time on the 10-minute consultation. *British Journal of General Practice* 2012; **62(596)**: 118–19.

41   Luft J, Ingham H. *Of Human Interaction*. Palo Alto: National Press, 1969.

42   Kirwan M, Armstrong D. Investigation of burnout in a sample of British general practitioners. *British Journal of General Practice* 1995; **45**: 259–60.

43   *Gold Standards Framework for Palliative Care*, www.goldstandardsframework. org.uk [accessed May 2012].

6 The applied knowledge

The condensed statements

This section of the book contains a summary of the core knowledge and skills of general practice described in the contextual statements and clinical examples of the RCGP Curriculum for Specialty Training for General Practice. For each statement, we have extracted the key educational content and packaged it into four easy-to-understand sections, as described on Table 6.1.

Table 6.1

Sections within each condensed statement	
The condensed knowledge	This contains the core items of knowledge contained in the statement's knowledge base (not all statements have this section)
The condensed skills	This contains the key skills described in the statement and our interpretation of how they apply to the topic or group of patients concerned
The condensed know-how	This contains the key applied knowledge extracted from the learning outcomes for the statement
The condensed resources	This contains a selection of useful educational resources for learning and teaching the statement

Our tips for learning and teaching

Throughout this chapter we have included a variety of useful tips and resources to help support the learning and teaching of each curriculum statement. Some of these are taken from the resources listed in the full statements and others are derived from other sources including the published literature and the advice of established trainers, course organisers and GP educationalists.

To the right-hand side of each item of knowledge or skill we have included boxes for you to tick or score. How you use these boxes depends on how you plan to use the book in your learning (Table 6.2, overleaf).

Table 6.2

Tick or score	
Tick ☑	You can use the condensed curriculum as a checklist, ticking each box when you have read the item concerned, or marking that you are confident that you have mastered the relevant item of knowledge, skill or know-how
Score	You can use 'The essential knowledge' as a *self-assessment confidence rating scale* by giving each item of knowledge, skill or know-how a score from **1–5**: **1** – I am not at all confident in this area of knowledge or ability **2** – I have some knowledge or ability here, but don't feel I am competent **3** – I am probably competent at this but would like to learn more **4** – I feel confident my current knowledge or ability is competent **5** – I am simply awesome at this! This process can help you identify the knowledge and skills you feel least confident about and assist in setting priorities for planning your learning. First, focus on addressing the items that you scored '**1**', then move on to those marked '**2**' and so on. You may wish to repeat this exercise over time as your expertise progresses ('spiral learning'). It is advisable to ask a trainer or mentor who has observed your performance to review your scores in order to check that your subjective assessment is a true reflection of your abilities. If there is more than 1 point of disagreement between you and your trainer over a particular item, discuss why this might be.

Table 6.3

Index of condensed statements

			Page
Core Statement	1.0	*Being a General Practitioner* – this is explored in detail in Chapter 5 'The core curriculum'.	**77**
Contextual statements	2.01	*The GP Consultation in Practice*	**136**
	2.02	*Patient Safety and Quality of Care*	**143**
	2.03	*The GP in the Wider Professional Environment*	**151**
	2.04	*Enhancing Professional Knowledge*	**156**
Clinical examples	3.01	*Healthy People: promoting health and preventing disease*	**165**
	3.02	*Genetics in Primary Care*	**172**
	3.03	*Care of Acutely Ill People*	**178**
	3.04	*Care of Children and Young People*	**187**
	3.05	*Care of Older Adults*	**195**
	3.06	*Women's Health*	**200**
	3.07	*Men's Health*	**208**
	3.08	*Sexual Health*	**214**
	3.09	*End-of-Life Care*	**223**
	3.10	*Care of People with Mental Health Problems*	**228**
	3.11	*Care of People with Intellectual Disability*	**235**
	3.12	*Cardiovascular Health*	**240**
	3.13	*Digestive Health*	**245**
	3.14	*Care of People Who Misuse Drugs and Alcohol*	**250**
	3.15	*Care of People with ENT, Oral and Facial Problems*	**256**
	3.16	*Care of People with Eye Problems*	**262**
	3.17	*Care of People with Metabolic Problems*	**267**
	3.18	*Care of People with Neurological Problems*	**273**
	3.19	*Respiratory Health*	**278**
	3.20	*Care of People with Musculoskeletal Problems*	**284**
	3.21	*Care of People with Skin Problems*	**292**

Wide-ranging curriculum resources

There are numerous educational resources available to GP trainees, trainers and established GPs that support learning and teaching across the breadth of general practice. We have identified a handful of resources that offer a wide range of material relevant to large areas of the curriculum. To avoid repeating these resources in every condensed statement, they are listed here as wide-ranging curriculum resources.

Table 6.4

RCGP curriculum resources	
The RCGP website, www.rcgp.org.uk	Provides a wealth of information on the curriculum, GP training and education, and MRCGP assessments, plus news on educational courses and events. The RCGP website also enables College members and Associates-in-Training to gain free access to a range of popular subscription-only journals including: • *British Medical Journal* (BMJ) • *British Journal of General Practice* (BJGP) • *Education for Primary Care* • *Evidence-Based Medicine* • *Journal of the American Medical Association* (JAMA) • *The Lancet*
The RCGP Online Learning Environment, www.elearning.rcgp. org.uk	Offers RCGP online updates, courses and certifications for GPs on a wide range of primary care topics. Also includes the Personal Education Planning (PEP) tools, which enable you to assess your learning needs and map them against the GP curriculum
e-GP: e-Learning for General Practice, www.e-GP.org	A large programme of RCGP e-learning modules on many curriculum topics, free to NHS healthcare workers
***InnovAiT*, www.rcgp.org.uk/ innovait**	The RCGP journal for Associates-in-Training that covers the RCGP curriculum and provides educational articles, news and views on a variety of GP training topics

Table 6.5

Other useful educational resources	
BetterTesting, www.bettertesting.org.uk	A question-and-answer format website with information about requesting laboratory tests
BMJ Learning, www.learning.bmj.com	Online learning from the BMJ group – contains some free modules but a subscription is required for many
NHS Choices, www.nhs.uk	While predominantly aimed at patients, there are lots of useful areas for clinicians, including a summary of the National Service Frameworks (NSFs) and strategies (www.nhs.uk/NHSEngland/NSF/Pages/Nationalserviceframeworks.aspx)
Healthtalkonline, www.healthtalkonline.org	Read, watch and listen to patients and their carers discussing their experiences of health and illness
Doctors.net, www.doctors.net.uk	Offers a range of educational resources for doctors, including a wide range of accredited learning modules on general practice topics
GPnotebook, www.gpnotebook.co.uk	A popular and accessible online encyclopaedia of medicine that is a particularly useful resource for learning the knowledge base contained within the curriculum. It also offers GP Notebook Educational Modules ('GEMS'), which allow learners to test themselves on important GP topics
NHS Evidence, www.evidence.nhs.uk	Search engine for health and social care professionals, providing access to evidence-based health information. Contains numerous resources of interest to GP learners
National Institute for Health and Clinical Excellence (NICE), www.nice.org.uk	Develops many evidence-based clinical practice guidelines for the NHS in England and Wales
Patient.co.uk, www.patient.co.uk	Website containing a large amount of clinical information, patient information leaflets, self-help information and contact details of relevant organisations
Scottish Intercollegiate Guidelines Network (SIGN), www.sign.ac.uk	Develops many evidence-based clinical practice guidelines for the NHS in Scotland

Statement 2.01: *The GP Consultation in Practice*

Effective communication and consultation skills are at the heart of good general practice. A GP should be able to communicate clearly, sensitively and effectively, be committed to patient-centred medicine and have a clear understanding of what makes a good consultation and how it is achieved.

GPs, in common with all health professionals, must act in accordance with the ethical principles set out in professional codes of conduct. Ethical decision making and behaviour require the application and interpretation of these principles within the specific context of general practice, taking into account the perspectives and values of all involved. In all aspects of practice, GPs need to be able to justify their decisions with reference to both the clinical evidence and the moral and other values that inform them.

As consulting is so central to being a GP, many of the skills and attitudes required are described in the core areas of competence (see Chapter 5, 'The core curriculum').

The condensed skills

		☑ **or score** (1–5)
Consultation skills	Developing consultation skills typically associated with good doctor–patient communication, including:	
	• focusing your history and examination to help formulate a diagnosis, rule out serious illness and manage uncertainty	
	• adopting a non-judgemental approach	
	• adapting your approach as necessary to meet the needs and expectation of the patient (including working with interpreters)	
	• sharing information with patients in order to inform and educate them	
	• communicating with patients from diverse backgrounds and providing information in ways that help people to exercise their individual rights, including making effective use of interpreting and communications support services	

		☑ **or score (1–5)**
Consultation skills	• explaining risks and benefits in a meaningful way and offering patients evidence-based health choices	
	• communicating and consulting effectively and safely via telephone and email	
IM&T skills	Using the computer in a patient-centred consultation and keeping accurate, legible and contemporaneous patient records	
	Making effective use of the practice records system	
Moral reasoning skills	Considering the ethical dimension of every healthcare encounter	
	Resolving opposing values and choosing an appropriate course of action, such as balancing conflicting duties to two patients who are members of the same family	
Negotiation skills	Negotiating effectively with patients, relatives, carers and colleagues to develop an understanding of the problem and a shared and appropriate decision on its management (patient empowerment)	
	Using techniques to limit consultation length when appropriate	
Reflective skills	Undertaking self-appraisal through reflective logs and video recordings of consultations, and identifying learning needs from these; recognising, monitoring and managing emotions arising from the consultation	
	Recognising the limits of your abilities and expertise, and factors that may affect these	
	Recognising personal values and how these influence decision making and the ability to clarify and justify personal ethics	
Team-working skills	Communicating with, delegating to, managing and supporting colleagues and staff	
	Valuing people's beliefs and preferences, and actively promoting equality and addressing discrimination	

Continued over

		☑ **or score (1–5)**
Resource management	Using time and resources effectively during the consultation	
	Referring appropriately and using healthcare resources prudently	

The condensed know-how

	☑ **or score (1–5)**
The interrelation between a patient, his or her illness and others affected by his or her illness (including carers)	
How consulting behaviour, attitudes, cultural (and other) values and decision making may vary with age, gender, ethnicity, the social background of the patient and his or her current health state/phase of disease (e.g. entering the terminal phase of an illness)	
Common models of the consultation and how these models can be used to shape future consulting behaviour. **Tip:** *The common consultation models are summarised on p. 140*	
Models of the process by which patients decide to consult, and how this can affect consulting outcomes. **Tip:** *Helman's 'folk model of illness' (1981)[1] and Becker and Maiman's 'health belief model' (1975)[2] are relevant to this*	
How the doctor's agenda may conflict with the patient's or relative's agenda (e.g. QOF targets, evidence-based medicine, public health responsibilities, child safeguarding). **Tip:** *Always remember the central tenet of GP consulting: discover the patient's ideas, concerns and expectations[3]*	
Roles and expertise of colleagues and other primary healthcare team members	
How clinical coding systems are used and their role in effective record keeping. **Tip:** *Find out about Read codes and SNOMED codes*	

	☑ **or score (1–5)**
Resources and knowledge to support patient education and information sharing, the role of expert patients. **Tip:** *For info on expert patients go to: www.expertpatients.co.uk*	
How co-morbidity or disease progression may affect decision-making capacity in a patient and the steps that can be taken to maximise capacity. **Tip:** *Familiarise yourself with your duties in relation to the Mental Capacity Act 2005 and the Deprivation of Liberty Safeguards Assessments 2010*	
Methods of making timely and appropriate referrals (e.g. two-week wait or other local pathways)	
Inter-professional boundaries of clinical responsibility and confidentiality. **Tip:** *Review the six Caldicott principles* [4]	
Understanding the importance of continuity of care and long-term relationships with a patient and his or her family	
Evidence-based medicine – its role in management and referral decisions, and its limitations (including, for some patients, approaching their health/illness in a non-scientific way)	
Health promotion in the consultation, including educating patients on how to 'navigate' the healthcare system	
Ethical issues in the consultation relating to confidentiality, gaining meaningful consent for treatment (including the issues in patients who lack capacity), resolving conflicts of values, the extent to which patients choose to exercise their autonomy, being truthful and promoting justice	
Guidance on consent and confidentiality in the particular context of primary care. **Tip:** *Review the GMC's guidance on confidentiality*	

The condensed resources

The following table condenses six well-known consultation models:

Stott and Davis (1979)[5] – exceptional potential in each consultation	**Neighbour (1987)[6] – five-checkpoint model**
• Managing the presenting complaint • Managing ongoing problems • Opportunistic health promotion • Modifying health-seeking behaviour	• Connecting • Summarising • Handover • Safety-netting • Housekeeping
Pendleton et al. (1984, 2003)[3] – seven-tasks model	**Tuckett et al. (1985)[7] – meeting of two experts**
• Define the reason for the patient's attendance (ideas, concerns and expectations) • Consider other problems • Choose appropriate action • Share understanding with the patient • Involve the patient in management decisions • Use time and resources well • Establish and maintain the doctor–patient relationship	• The consultation is a meeting between two experts • Doctors are experts in medicine • Patients are experts in their own illnesses • Shared understanding is the aim • Doctors should seek to understand the patient's beliefs • Doctors should address explanations in terms of the patient's belief system
Stewart et al. (1995, 2003)[8] – patient-centred clinical method	**Calgary–Cambridge observation guide (1996)[9] – stages of a consultation**
• Exploring both the disease and the illness experience • Understanding the whole person • Finding common ground • Incorporating prevention and health promotion • Enhancing the doctor–patient relationship • Being realistic (with time and resources)	• Initiating the session • Gathering information • Building the relationship • Explanation and planning • Closing the session

A large collection of printable information leaflets suitable for UK patients is available at: www.patient.co.uk.

The following methods are useful for developing consultation skills:

- learn a number of consultation models (Roger Neighbour's 'five-checkpoint model' from *The Inner Consultation*[6] is insightful for everyday consulting)

- video your consultations – and force yourself to review them!

- analyse consultations with a trainer or mentor. The MRCGP consultation observation tool (COT) has been designed for this purpose (see Chapter 4, 'Succeeding at the MRCGP'). Alternatively, try 'consultation mapping' (www.gp-training.net)

- the Calgary–Cambridge model[10] is a useful framework for exploring new consultation techniques

- role-play with actors or colleagues (remember: 'no pain, no gain!')

- ask patients to give candid feedback at the end of the consultation

- sit in with an experienced GP and conduct joint surgeries with several GPs.

Below is a list of some of the textbooks and publications that have been influential in the development of GP consulting skills. They are worth a read. (A more extensive list is available in the full curriculum statement.)

- Berne E. *Games People Play*. London: Penguin, 1964.

- Goleman D. *Emotional Intelligence*. London: Bloomsbury, 1996.

- Neighbour R. *The Inner Consultation*. Lancaster: MTP, 1987.

- Pendleton D, Schofield T, Tate P, Havelock P. *The New Consultation: developing doctor–patient communication*. Oxford: Radcliffe Medical Press, 2003.

- Stott NC, Davis RH. The exceptional potential in each primary care consultation. *Journal of the Royal College of General Practitioners* 1979; **29**: 201–5.

- Tate P. *The Doctor's Communication Handbook* (4th edn). Oxford: Radcliffe Medical Press, 2002.

- Usherwood T. *Understanding the Consultation*. Buckingham: Open University Press, 1999.

The 'big four' ethical principles form a useful basic theoretical framework for considering ethical issues in the consultation:

Table 6.6

Four key ethical principles	
Beneficence	**Non-maleficence**
Doing good	Doing no harm
Autonomy	**Justice**
Acting in accordance with an individual's right to be free, independent and self-directing	Acting in accordance with the principles of truth, reason, fairness and the law

Statement 2.02: *Patient Safety and Quality of Care*

GPs don't work alone but within teams and systems of care, and are in a particularly strong position to positively influence the safety culture within their practices.

Addressing the safety of patients systematically across both the practice and wider NHS is an essential part of the GP's role. To do this, GPs need to make sure that their practice has good systems in place to monitor the safety and quality of care that they provide and to respond to near misses and significant events. This involves leadership, team-working and good information systems. The knowledge and application of risk assessment tools must become part of a GP's core set of skills and, whenever change occurs in their working environment, GPs should assess the risks of this change and plan accordingly.

GPs increasingly need to be able to demonstrate that they keep up to date and are fit to practise, and can account for the standard of care they are providing. Every GP must understand the principles of clinical governance and use them in his or her everyday professional practice. The main aim of clinical governance is to improve the quality and accountability of health care, to identify and respond to poor practice, and to create a supportive culture with good teamwork, underpinned by clinical audit.

The condensed skills

		☑ **or score** **(1–5)**
Communication skills	Communicating openly, listening and taking patients' concerns seriously, and telling patients fully, honestly and compassionately about incidents and errors when they occur	
Reflective skills	Identifying the limitations of your own skills in risk management (as well as more widely) and knowing when the risk assessment professionals should be called upon, being aware of your accountability as a GP	
Risk assessment skills	Carrying out a risk assessment using a risk matrix. **Tip:** *The Health and Safety Executive (HSE) website has a useful guide on carrying out a risk assessment: www.hse.gov.uk*	

Continued over

		☑ **or score** **(1–5)**
Team-working skills	Sharing and implementing lessons within the team from the analysis of patient safety incidents. Giving and receiving feedback effectively. **Tip:** *Familiarise yourself with the Pendleton rules*[3] *for giving effective feedback (see Chapter 3, 'Learning and Teaching the Curriculum')*	
IM&T skills	Using the practice clinical system for tasks such as prescribing, entering clinical data, processing pathology results and referrals. This includes using:	
	• templates for the management of chronic disease and assessing risk	
	• recall systems within the practice to the benefit of patient care	
	• inter-agency systems such as pathology links and GP-to-GP record transfer	
	• the computer in the consultation while maintaining rapport with the patient	
	• NHS electronic booking systems (e.g. 'Choose and Book') to tailor healthcare provision to the needs of the individual patient	
	• ePortfolio tools for training, appraisal and revalidation	
Audit skills	Completing an eight-stage clinical audit. **Tip:** *The eight-stage audit process is shown below*	
	Completing Significant Event Audit	
EBM skills	Locating (and implementing) information about standards and clinical guidelines	
	Undertaking critical appraisal of practice performance data (e.g. referrals, prescribing)	
Change management skills	Illustrating how a change in behaviour or systems can influence patient safety by planning and implementing a change in the practice. **Tip:** *Review the PDSA cycle (plan–do–study–act)*[11]	

	☑ **or score** **(1–5)**
Learning skills Developing and maintaining an approach to continuing learning and quality improvement	

The condensed know-how

	☑ **or score** **(1–5)**
The definition of clinical governance, local clinical governance arrangements, current clinical governance guidelines and understanding of the role and responsibilities of a practice clinical governance lead	
How organisations and individuals can learn to be vigilant for patient safety incidents and how a change in clinical behaviour and/or practice systems influences patient safety and the impact of the GP's working environment on risk. **Tip:** *Participate in risk management meetings and discussions in the practice and consider how to develop a 'safety culture'* **Tip:** *Keep a log diary of consecutive consultations for one day a month to try to identify actual or potential patient safety issues* **Tip:** *Read about Situational Awareness Theory (e.g. Reason's 'Three Buckets' model)* [12]	
How analysis of patient safety incidents and near misses can be applied prospectively to improve systems and enhance performance (using the principles of 'improvement methodology' to facilitate change)	
The basic principles of risk assessment and the elements of an appropriate infrastructure for clinical and non-clinical risk management are: • creating a culture that is open, honest and fair	
• policies and systems that state the actions that staff should take following an incident	
• individual roles and accountability	
• the mechanism of investigating errors	
• support for patients, family and staff	

Continued over

	☑ **or score (1–5)**

- staff training including shared learning and continual incremental improvement.

Tip: *Identify the systems and processes set up in your practice to manage risk and compare these systems with those in the practices of your colleagues*

Tip: *Consider the various different 'risk areas' in your practice – e.g. clinical negligence, patient and staff health and safety issues, environmental risks, financial risks, complaints handling*

Tip: *Risk management tools are available on the medical indemnity organisation and HPA websites*

Clinical risk reduction and detection of adverse events involves:

- the basic principles of human error

- common medical errors

- the causes of delayed referrals

- recording significant events

- reporting adverse incidents.

Tip: *Familiarise yourself with the yellow-card system for reporting adverse drug events. Look in the back of the BNF or at: www.yellowcard.gov.uk for more details*

Medical device management principles.

Significant Event Analysis (SEA) involves:

- understanding the triggers for performing an SEA or root cause analysis

- considering the rationale for participation of the multidisciplinary team in SEA and reasons for the inclusion or exclusion of different team members

	☑ **or score** **(1–5)**

- identifying methods of feeding back fairly to colleagues and implementing solutions to reduce the risk of harm (including appropriate learning)

- discussing how to embed any lessons learnt in the practice's working processes and systems

- identifying other patient services that may be affected by the same issues in future and how to share learning more widely.

Tip: *Write up an SEA from a patient seen during the general practice period of training. Reflect on the learning and consider whether reporting locally or nationally would be appropriate. Identify the measures that the practice takes to ensure that significant events are dealt with fairly and that the appropriate learning and action take place*

Take steps to facilitate safer multi-professional working with:

- other practice team members

- community teams (e.g. pharmacists, nurses, health visitors, matrons and case managers, and other community roles)

- secondary care

- social services and other non-medical professionals.

Tip: *Consider a patient pathway in which a number of different professionals have been involved. Reflect on the safety issues arising from the interfaces between providers and the ways in which these risks can be reduced (e.g. quality of communication, referral letters, and handovers)*

Quality improvement systems:

- the general principles, methods and concepts of quality assurance

- NHS quality improvement systems at national and local levels

- involvement of patients and the local community to assist in service planning/improvement (including vulnerable and excluded populations)

- methods for ascertaining the views of patients (e.g. through patient participation groups)

- describing when an improvement project would help patient care and how to evaluate it

Continued over

	☑ **or score (1–5)**
• models of change management	
• methods of obtaining feedback (qualitative and quantitative)	
How to facilitate patient access to his or her medical record, the relevant rules and to enhance patient understanding of privacy and the consent issues concerning the shared electronic health record	
Understanding of how the NHS complaints system works and how to deal with and learn from complaints. **Tip:** *Find out about the role of the Patient Advice and Liaison Service (PALS): www.pals.nhs.uk*	
Understand the financial and legal frameworks in which health care is given at a practice level including the various codes of practice (professional, regulatory, NHS and legal). **Tip:** *Read the General Medical Council's* Good Medical Practice [13] *and compare with the RCGP's* Good Medical Practice for General Practitioners [14]	
Understand the ethical tensions inherent in governance processes and resource allocation decisions	
How patient groups may be put at increased risk or mishap or health inequality by virtue of their particular characteristics, such as language, literacy, culture and health beliefs. **Tip:** *Consider how to improve access for 'hard to reach' groups*	
The issues around poor clinical performance: • why variation in clinical care occurs	
• methods of assessment and management, performance indicators, local and national procedures	
• whistle blowing and raising concerns about colleagues – when and how. Support for poorly performing doctors	
The inter-relationship between clinical governance, appraisal and revalidation (including the requirements, systems and resources for revalidation)	

	☑ **or score** **(1–5)**
The use (and abuse) of information for benchmarking purposes to analyse doctor and practice performance, compare practices and inform future healthcare agendas. **Tip:** *Connecting for Health is the government body responsibility for NHS IT infrastructure: www.connectingforhealth.nhs.uk*	
Ethical and legal issues around the sharing of local or centrally held electronic patient information (with the patient and with other professionals). **Tip:** *Find out about the Freedom of Information, Access to Medical Reports and Data Protection Acts*	

The condensed resources

- The National Reporting and Learning Service enables confidential reporting of patient safety incidents in England and Wales: www.nrls.npsa.nhs.uk.

- The Medicines and Healthcare products Regulatory Agency is the government agency responsible for ensuring that medicines and medical devices are safe. Its website contains lots of information on patient safety as well as safety warnings, alerts and how to report safety concerns: www.mhra.gov.uk.

- The Health and Safety Executive provides useful information on health and safety issues, and performing risk assessment: www.hse.gov.uk.

- Your local Clinical Governance Support Team can provide information, guidance and assistance in successfully implementing clinical governance.

- NHS Quality Improvement Scotland (NHS QIS) is the lead organisation for improving the quality of health care in Scotland: www.nhshealthquality.org.

The eight-stage clinical audit cycle

1 Describe the reason for choice of audit, considering the potential for change and relevance of the audit to the practice.

2 Identify the audit criteria, ensuring the criteria chosen are relevant to the audit subject and are justified by relevant evidence.

3 Set the audit standards; this involves setting appropriate targets and a suitable time scale.

4 Prepare and plan the audit, recording evidence of teamwork and discussion where appropriate.

5 Complete the first data collection, comparing the results against the standards.

6 Implement the changes to be evaluated, with examples described.

7 Complete the second data collection and compare the results with the first data collection and the standards.

8 Describe the conclusions, including any barriers to change and a summary of the issues learned.

The seven domains of 'Standards for Better Health' used in England are:[15]

- Safety

- Clinical and Cost-Effectiveness

- Governance

- Patient Focus

- Accessible and Responsive Care

- Care Environment and Amenities

- Public Health.

Statement 2.03: *The GP in the Wider Professional Environment*

GPs need the skills to manage their practice or organisation effectively and also in the development and organisation of services and Primary Care Organisations. Working with patients, GPs need to lead changes in service delivery to improve population health outcomes and quality of care.

The condensed skills

		☑ or score (1–5)
Staff development skills	Participating in the recruitment of staff, their development and training (including appraisal)	
	Motivating staff and understanding the role of team dynamics in this process. **Tip:** *Maslow's Hierarchy of Needs*[16] *and McClelland's motivational needs theory*[17] *are useful models for understanding what motivates different people*	
Team-working skills	Understanding your preference for roles within a team and working as part of an effective team (including leading it). **Tip:** *Familiarise yourself with the Belbin team roles*[18]	
	Bringing individuals and groups together to achieve goals, maintaining team focus and managing team dynamics. **Tip:** *Identify a project that you can contribute to in your practice (e.g. setting up a new chronic disease clinic)*	
	Actively seeking the views of others and taking account of their needs, feeling, values and expertise. **TIP:** Organise and chair a practice meeting	
	Gaining the trust and support of colleagues. **Tip:** *The Multi-Source Feedback (MSF) tool of the MRCGP Workplace-based Assessment tests this skill*	
	Negotiating effectively with colleagues, staff and patients	

Continued over

		☑ **or score** **(1–5)**
Team-working skills	Delegating effectively. **Tip:** *Delegated tasks should be SMART: Specific, Measurable, Agreed, Realistic and Time-bound*	
Communication skills	Adopting strategies for effective communication within practice organisations. **Tip:** *Consider which type of meetings and other communication strategies are used in your practice. How reliable and effective are they?*	
Self-awareness skills	Being aware of your capabilities and values, strengths and limitations, and how stress and emotions affect you	
	Obtaining, analysing and acting on personal feedback from a variety of sources	
Leadership skills	Understanding the principles of leadership in the NHS. **Tip:** *Familiarise yourself with the NHS Medical Leadership Competency Framework (available at: www.institute.nhs.uk)*	
Service development skills	Placing patients at the centre of improving organisational performance and the quality of health care delivered by your practice. **Tip:** *Find out how to perform a SWOT analysis (Strengths, Weaknesses, Opportunities, Threats)*	
	Involving patients and the wider healthcare team in gathering information about healthcare needs and service improvements	
	Supporting development of services that respect diversity but are tailored to patient need	
	Adopting and disseminating models of good practice	
	Understanding the processes of quality improvement and change, and engaging positively with change	
	Applying quality improvement methodologies	

The condensed know-how

	☑ or score (1–5)
The roles of the various members of the primary care team. **Tip:** *Towards the start of your GP placement, make a list of all the people who work in your primary care team and their respective roles*	
Possible management structures of a practice, including how decisions are made and how responsibilities are distributed, and how this varies in different settings (e.g. rural, inner city, urban, academic, dispensing). **Tip:** *Try mapping out your practice's management structure. Compare it with other local practices. If you can't easily map it out, what does that imply?*	
The business and financial aspects of a practice, such as sources of income and expenditure, management of funding, use of premises, marketing, and the interpretation of accounts and factors affecting profitability. **Tip:** *Information on practice finances is available at: www.gponline.com/ medeconomics*	
The various NHS contractual arrangements for general practice (e.g. General Medical Services [GMS], Personal Medical Services [PMS], etc.) and the key features of these contractual agreements (e.g. global sum, QOF, enhanced services). **Tip:** *Information on the various GP contracts (GMS, PMS, etc.) and other relevant practice management issues can be found on the Department of Health (DH) website (www.dh.gov.uk) and the British Medical Association website (www.bma.org.uk)*	
The role of primary care in the context of the wider NHS and how health services are managed locally, regionally and nationally	
Local factors – the impact of the local community on your workplace, on patient care, on the structure of the local healthcare system and on its economic limitations	
The influence of local, regional and national health priorities, policies, guidelines, resources and facilities on the delivery of care. The important national and local strategies for health care and the current UK priorities and guidelines that influence service design and delivery. **Tip:** *The health white paper* Equity and Excellence: liberating the NHS *is available at: www.dh.gov.uk*	

Continued over

	☑ or score (1–5)
The role of local government and social services and the private and third sector in health. Working with these agencies to improve population health outcomes	
The variety of ways in which health care and health promotion may be delivered in the community (e.g. nurse-led clinics, case management) and how variation in resources and facilities may affect the delivery of health care	
An overview of clinically led commissioning – the GP's role as commissioner in England, the process of how services are commissioned and the conflicts of interest that might arise in the commissioning and provision of services. **Tip:** *The RCGP's Centre for Commissioning provides educational resources to help GPs to develop commissioning skills*	
Ways to establish the expectations that patients, carers and families have of their practice and local primary care services. **Tip:** *Find out if your practice has a patient participation group (PPG) and consider other ways of obtaining patient feedback*	
The duties, rights and responsibilities of a GP as an employer and the fundamentals of employment law including equal opportunities, recruitment practices and workplace anti-discrimination legislation. **Tip:** *This is a good topic for a tutorial with the practice manager. Also review your practice's employment policies and/or staff handbook*	
Procedures, policies and legislation appertaining to equality and diversity, including national law and international conventions relating to: ● human rights (including children) ● equality ● anti-discriminatory practices ● mental health ● complaints and issue resolution ● employment ● disability **Tip:** *Talk to your practice manager about the steps your practice has taken to comply with the Equality Act (with respect to both patients and staff)*	

	☑ **or score** **(1–5)**
The health and occupational safety responsibilities of a GP (either as an employer or co-worker). **Tip:** *See the condensed statement 2.02:* Patient Safety and Quality of Care	
Ethical aspects relating to management and leadership in primary care (e.g. use of resources, rationing, involving the public and patients in decision making, conflicts of interest, balancing the needs of the individual GP, the practice, the individual patient and the health needs of the local community)	
The issues around whistle-blowing and where to get advice and support	
The environmental impact of services and the need for sustainable use of resources. The impact of climate change on health and how the GP can contribute to reduction in CO_2 production and the principles of co-benefits	
The wider social responsibilities of doctors in relation to the environmental contributors to the social determinants of health and in becoming altruistically involved in societal issues that would benefit from their input. Actively seeking to inform and influence decision makers	

The condensed resources

- First Practice Management provides a range of resources to support medical practice managers: www.firstpracticemanagement. co.uk.

- A collection of generic educational resources on teamwork, leadership and business skills is available at: www.businessballs.com.

Statement 2.04: *Enhancing Professional Knowledge*

GPs need to understand the principles of evidence-based medicine and how to apply these to individual patients and carers, to the practice and to the wider healthcare system. This requires the ability to search for evidence from a wide range of online and real-world sources, interpret and appraise this evidence, and then apply it to practice. A basic understanding of primary care research is also a requirement for every GP.

Teaching, mentoring and supervision are also core activities of general practice and, at some stage, every GP will have some form of teaching, mentoring or supervisory role. Many of the skills needed for effective consulting with patients are similar to the skills required for effective teaching and a learner-centred approach is required. GP trainees are likely to be increasingly involved in teaching in the future, in educational activities involving other trainees and within their multidisciplinary teams.

The condensed knowledge

		☑ or score (1–5)
Basic statistics	Absolute risk (AR) and absolute risk reduction (ARR)	
	Hazard ratio (HR)	
	Incidence and prevalence	
	Number needed to harm (NNH) and number needed to treat (NNT)	
	Odds and odds ratio (OR)	
	Pre- and post-test probability	
	Positive predictive value (PPV) and negative predictive value (NPV)	
	Relative risk (RR) and relative risk reduction (RRR)	
	Specificity and sensitivity	

		☑ **or score** **(1–5)**
Critical appraisal	Appropriateness of prospective and retrospective studies	
	Bias, inclusion and exclusion criteria, and representativeness of samples	
	Common tests used to analyse parametric data (e.g. awareness of t-tests, analysis of variance, multiple regression) and non-parametric data (e.g. awareness of chi-squared, Mann–Whitney U tests)	
	Confidence intervals, probability and correlation coefficients	
	Methods used to validate qualitative research (e.g. triangulation, saturation)	
	Reliability, validity and generalisability of findings	
Research methodologies	Case-control studies	
	Cohort studies	
	Interviews, focus groups and questionnaires	
	Meta-analysis	
	Narrative-based research	
	Pilot studies	
	Primary care research networks	
	Qualitative research	
	Quantitative research	
	Randomised controlled trials	
	Research databases used in general practice (e.g. Q Research)	
	Systematic reviews	

Continued over

The condensed skills

		☑ or score (1–5)
Communication skills	Communicating risks and benefits in a way that is meaningful to patients	
Consulting skills	Enhancing patient concordance with evidence-based lifestyle and therapeutic interventions	
	Explaining the rationale for an evidence-based approach, taking into account the patient's aims, priorities and values	
	Managing uncertainty through evidence-based practice, explaining the lack of evidence when necessary and why this has arisen	
Evidence-based practice skills	Searching, identifying, evaluating, interpreting and applying best evidence and offering healthcare choices based on this evidence in an objective manner, tailored to the problem and to the preferences and needs of the patient	
Adult learning skills	Carrying out an educational needs analysis and setting your own learning objectives based on your clinical and professional experiences. **Tip:** *Chapter 3, 'Learning and teaching the curriculum', contains information on how to do this*	
Feedback skills	Giving constructive feedback to a colleague as a teacher or mentor	
IM&T skills	Making good use of information management and technology in both individual and group teaching. **Tip:** *Every training practice should have access to a projector or large screen for presentations*	
Prescribing skills	Effective and evidence-based primary care prescribing, following the GMC's principles of good prescribing	
Presentation skills	Delivering a presentation clearly and effectively, identifying the needs of the audience, tailoring the presentation to those needs and encouraging active involvement. **Tip:** *Give a short presentation to your training group; ask them to give you feedback*	

	☑ or score (1–5)
Teaching and mentoring skills	Planning and structuring a teaching episode (activity) appropriately for the learners concerned and facilitating the learning of a small group.
	Tip: *Training programmes should include a self-directed element to help trainees develop these skills*
	The ability to ask for, organise, receive and also give forms of mentorship and supervision appropriate to each career stage
Research skills **Tip:** *Look at the Centre for Evidence-Based Medicine's website for tips on how to develop these skills: www.cebm.net*	Evaluating ethical issues and the need to have projects approved through research governance committees
	Implementing change in clinical practice
	Prioritising relevant information
	Problem framing

The condensed know-how

	☑ or score (1–5)
Reliable sources of the best possible evidence to base decisions and to inform patients of the 'best possible' way to navigate the healthcare system	
Basic statistics and how to evaluate an original scientific paper, a review paper and an evidence-based guideline. **Tip:** *there are lots of books on basic statistics. Or look at: www.cebm.net*	
Factors affecting the efficacy of evidence-based interventions:	
• concordance with therapeutic aims	
• continuity of care and a long-term relationship	
• the role of the doctor–patient relationship.	

Continued over

	☑ **or score** **(1–5)**
Tip: *A combination of evidence-based treatments is not necessarily an evidence-based approach in itself. Interactions between the various interventions may affect efficacy*	
Understanding that patients may wish to self-manage based on their own interpretation of scientific knowledge and awareness of the scarcity of evidence derived from a patient's perspective. **Tip:** *Consider the relative merits of quantitative and qualitative research*	
The application of multi-morbidity research and the limitations of evidence in the elderly or in patients with complex co-morbidity, as much evidence excludes these patients	
Consider psychosocial factors, intellectual disability, vulnerability and cultural background when taking an evidence-based approach (on both an individual and a population level)	
The issue of health inequalities when applying evidence to minorities and awareness that evidence may not reflect the diversity of your local population. **Tip::** *Always check to see if the population in a study is applicable to your own practice's population*	
Understanding that health economic and resource allocation data support the recommendations on which many treatments are offered (e.g. NICE guidance)	
The limitations of separating scientific and non-scientific approaches to health and the issues arising when patients differ from their doctors in the value they attach to medical evidence. **Tip:** *A patient's objectives in a consultation are often driven by his or her values, although the solutions a GP can offer are often 'value-neutral', or based on the medical profession's values. For example, an evidence-based guideline for diagnosing headache is unlikely to offer much comfort to an anxious patient whose relative recently died of a stroke*	
The difference between research and clinical audit	
The benefits and limitations of local healthcare reviews and surveys	

	☑ **or score** **(1–5)**
The impact of local prescribing incentives and dealing with conflicts of interest	
The research process:	
● develop a research question	
● identify appropriate methods from a range of designs	_____
● be able to draw up a questionnaire	_____
● demonstrate basic quantitative and qualitative data-analysis skills	_____
● draw appropriate conclusions	_____
● summarise results.	_____
Tip: *The RCGP website contains information for GPs interested in carrying out research: www.rcgp.org.uk/research*	
How to provide patients involved in research with full information and obtain informed consent	
Ethical considerations in research, including the role of ethics committees and the patient's right to choose whether or not to participate or to accept new interventions. **Tip:** *Consider how the principles of informed consent and patient autonomy applied to your recent consultations*	
Confidentiality, research governance and Data Protection Act requirements. **Tip:** *The Information Commissioner provides advice and tools on the Data Protection Act: www.ico.gov.uk*	
The range of resources available from postgraduate and university departments. **Tip:** *Your local continuing professional development (CPD) tutor should be able to provide information on local academic resources*	
Principles of adult learning theory. **Tip:** *See Chapter 3, 'Learning and teaching the curriculum'*	

Continued over

	☑ **or score** **(1–5)**
The principles of a learner-centred approach to teaching, including needs analysis and individual learning styles and preferences.	
Tip: *Consider completing a learning style questionnaire to identify your learning preferences (e.g. Honey and Mumford,*[19] *which divides learners into theorists, activists, pragmatists and reflectors)*	
The benefits of inter-professional and multi-professional learning	
The nature and purpose of mentoring and clinical supervision, and the different forms of these (both formal and informal)	
The relationship between teaching and reflective practice. **Tip:** *Keep a reflective diary to record significant consultations*	
Ways of establishing a culture of teaching and learning within a practice and more broadly within the local healthcare community. **Tip:** *www.gp-training.net has more information on learning organisations*	
Models of teaching (didactic, Socratic, etc. [see Table 6.7])	

The condensed resources

- The web has many sources of evidence for use in general practice. Among the most useful are:
  - NHS Evidence: www.evidence.nhs.uk
  - The Cochrane Library: www.thecochranelibrary.com
  - The NICE guidelines: www.nice.org.uk
  - The SIGN guidelines: www.sign.ac.uk.
- Information on EBM, critical appraisal and statistics can be found here:
  - the Oxford Centre for Evidence-Based Medicine: www.cebm.net
  - the EBM journal *Bandolier* contains a glossary explaining key research terms: www.medicine.ox.ac.uk/bandolier/glossary.html
  - Trisha Greenhalgh's book *How to Read a Paper: the basics of evidence based medicine* (Blackwell Publishing, 2006) provides a useful introduction to evidence-based medicine.

- *e*-GP contains RCGP e-learning sessions on evidence-based practice (www.e-GP.org).

- The Honey and Mumford learning styles questionnaire is available from: www.peterhoney.com.

- The Myers–Briggs Personality Indicator is available from: www.myersbriggs.org.

- Chapter 3, 'Learning and teaching the curriculum', contains lots of information and advice relevant to this statement.

Developing teaching skills

GPs, as lifelong learners and educators, may become involved in leading a variety of educational activities throughout their career. These activities may include one-on-one tutorials, group teaching, seminars, workshops and presentations, all of which require different teaching styles and techniques. Developing a range of teaching styles can help educators engage more successfully with their learners and improve the effectiveness of the teaching. Successful educators develop the ability to choose from a wide range of teaching styles, according to the situation.

Table 6.7

Teaching methods and roles

Method	Process	Role of the teacher	Relevant authors
Didactic	Telling	Passing on knowledge	Many authors
Socratic	Questioning	Facilitating learning through awareness-raising questions	Neighbour 1992 [20]
Heuristic	Encouraging	Promoting learner autonomy and self-directed learning	Kolb 1984 [21] Knowles 1990 [22] Brookfield 1986 [23]
Counselling	Exploring	Encouraging self-awareness, self-discovery and reflective practice through exploring feelings and examining assumptions by using discussion and judicious challenge	Schön 1987 [24] Heron 1990 [25] Bolton 2001 [26]

Source: RCGP curriculum statement 2.04 *Enhancing Professional Knowledge*.

What is evidence-based practice?

The process of evidence-based practice has been described as follows:

- translation of uncertainty into answerable questions

- systematic retrieval of the best evidence available

- critical appraisal for validity, clinical relevance and applicability

- application of results in practice

- evaluation of performance (either at an individual or organisational level).

Source: Dawes M, Summerskill W, Glaziou P, *et al.*[27]

Statement 3.01: *Healthy People: promoting health and preventing disease*

GPs provide the link between individual health care and care for the local community. A GP must, therefore, understand the concepts of health, function and quality of life as well as models of disease. Good population health requires effective health promotion, health prevention and accessible healthcare services for all. Gaining a good understanding of health inequalities, and the strategies to address these, is an important aspect of GP training.

GPs must also develop the skills to help people to self-care and to support carers, via a range of approaches. This should be done as a partnership, recognising that patients, with their carers, should make the necessary choices and decisions, and take the actions themselves. During the consultation, there are many opportunities to promote health and aid the prevention of illness and long-term worklessness. The GP also plays a key leadership role in supporting health through the practice team and the community more widely.

The condensed knowledge

		☑ or score (1–5)
Health promotion	Causes of inequalities in health	
	Concepts of health, disease, health promotion and quality of life. **Tip:** *The WHO definition of health is available at: www.who.int/about/definition/en/print.html*	
	Concepts of incidence and prevalence. **Tip:** *These are defined in Chapter 5, 'The core curriculum'*	
	Factors associated with health and ill health from before birth to old age (e.g. housing, employment, education)	
	Principles of rehabilitation after illness or injury	
	Risk factors for childhood accidents, child abuse and neglect	
	Risk factors for disease associated with lifestyle choices (e.g. smoking, alcohol and substance misuse, accidents, diet, exercise, occupation, sexual behaviour)	

Continued over

		☑ **or score** **(1–5)**
Disease prevention	NHS disease prevention programmes and strategies, including:	
	● Childhood immunisation programme	_____
	Tip: *The DoH immunisation website is available at: www.immunisation.dh.gov.uk*	
	● Notifiable diseases	_____
	Tip: *A list of these is available on the Health Protection Agency (HPA) website at: www.hpa.org.uk*	
	● Population health surveillance systems	_____
	Tip: *Find out about the RCGP Weekly Returns Service*	
	● Screening programmes	_____
	Tip: *Information on NHS screening programmes can be found at: www.screening.nhs.uk and the specific cancer screening website is www.cancerscreening.nhs.uk*	_____
Healthcare services	Stages of the commissioning cycle for healthcare services:	
	● analyse and plan (identifying population needs and reviewing existing services)	_____
	● design new pathways (reviewing evidence and data to design integrated, locally tailored services)	_____
	● specify and procure (agreeing service outcomes, providers and contracts)	_____
	● deliver and improve (monitoring performance and improving quality of care)	_____
	Strategies to address inequalities in access to health care	_____

The condensed skills

		☑ or score (1–5)
Communication skills	Communicating the risks of unhealthy behaviours and the benefits of lifestyle change effectively to patients, carers and families, both in the practice and local community	
Consultation skills	Promoting health on an individual basis as part of the consultation and judging when a patient will be receptive, displaying tolerance and understanding of the patient's views on health promotion interventions	
	Skills for delivering 'brief interventions' in the consultation. **Tip:** *See clinical example 3.14* Care of People Who Misuse Drugs and Alcohol	
	Techniques for reaching a shared understanding with patients about their problems, their natural history and management, so that patients are empowered to look after their own health	
	Techniques for exploring ideas about health and work, explaining the long-term health benefits of work, supporting return to work after absence and reducing long-term worklessness	
	Strategies to minimise the impact of a patient's symptoms on his or her wellbeing, taking into account biopsychosocial factors	

The condensed know-how

	☑ or score (1–5)
The use of the practice list as a framework for providing diagnostic, therapeutic and preventive services to individuals and to the registered population and the limitations of this approach (e.g. for unregistered patients)	
The principles of health promotion and disease prevention strategies, and the scientific backgrounds of public health, epidemiology and preventive health care.	
Tip: *Visit the Bandolier evidence-based medicine website at www.medicine.ox.ac.uk/bandolier/glossary.html*	

Continued over

	☑ **or score** **(1–5)**
The impact of poverty, genetics, ethnicity, geography, culture, the workplace and local epidemiology on an individual and a local community's health	
The impact of inequalities and discrimination on health and the 'inverse care law', and the importance of involving the public and communities in improving health and reducing inequalities. **Tip:** *Tudor Hart, a GP, first described the inverse care law in 1971.*[28] *He has a website where you can read about his life and work as a GP in Wales at: www.juliantudorhart.org*	
The role of the GP and the primary healthcare team in contributing to health promotion activities in the community. **Tip:** *The NICE Public Health Guidance is available at: www.nice.org.uk/guidance/phg*	
The principles of immunisation and vaccination, the UK's immunisation programmes and the benefits and risks of immunisation. **Tip:** *The Green Book (Immunisation against Infectious Disease) is available on the DH website at: www.immunisation.dh.gov.uk/category/the-green-book*	
The benefits and risks of screening programmes, and how to interpret evidence about a screening programme and decide whether it is worthwhile – for individuals or for groups. **Tip:** *Review the Wilson and Junger criteria*[29] *for screening programmes (see below)*	
The role of the public health specialist and how and when to access specialist public health advice. *The Faculty of Public Health sets the standards for specialists in public health: www.fph.org.uk*	
The roles of the other professionals involved in population health, e.g. school nurses, health visitors and public health specialists. **Tip:** *Consider spending a day attached to some of these professionals*	
How to use available data to review and evaluate the health needs of the local population, compare these with that of other populations, and identify priorities for improvement	

	☑ **or score** **(1–5)**

The principles of health surveillance and how this helps with planning of health services, providing alerts for contingency planning and for monitoring the equitable distribution of health care.

Tip: *Current UK Child Health Surveillance policy can be found in* Health for All Children *(2006)*[30]

Tip: *Information about the UK influenza surveillance programme can be found on the HPA website at: www.hpa.org.uk*

The concept of risk, individual patient's risk factors and communicating risk to patients and the public.

Tip: *There is an excellent BMJ theme issue on this topic: BMJ 327 (7417) (www.bmj.com)*

The causes of potential tensions between the GP's health promotion and commissioning roles and the patient's own agenda and how to manage these

Behavioural change models (approaches to behavioural change and their relevance to health promotion and self-care).

Tip: *Review Prochaska and DiClemente's 'cycle of change' model*[31]

The evidence for the generally positive relationship between health and work and the negative impact of long-term worklessness on the health outcomes for patients and families. Specific issues around management of work and health/illness issues and the professionals involved in supporting patients at work.

Tip: *See www.healthyworkinguk.co.uk for advice and resources on 'fit notes' and helping patients to return to work*

Issues around people with a disability and the workplace

The concept of the hierarchy of evidence and the differences between evidence for interventions in healthy people and for those who are sick

Ethical issues in healthcare provision – including the universal right to health care, prioritisation, improving access, pre-symptomatic diagnosis, lifestyle choices and how this fits with your personal ethics

The condensed resources

- UK immunisation information and schedules can be found in the Green Book: www.immunisation.dh.gov.uk/category/the-green-book.

- Information about screening can be found on the UK screening portal: www.screening.nhs.uk.

- NICE offers a collection of public health guidelines at: www.nice.org.uk/guidance/phg.

- *e*-GP contains RCGP e-learning sessions on childhood vaccinations, health promotion, health inequalities, travel medicine and child safeguarding (www.e-GP.org).

- The RCGP online course 'Commissioning: what is it and what's my role?' introduces the basics of commissioning for GPs: www.elearning.rcgp.org.uk.

- The King's Fund is a charitable foundation that publishes reports and policy documents, many of which are relevant to issues around health inequalities: www.kingsfund.org.uk.

- The Picker Institute works to improve patient experiences of health care: www.pickereurope.org.

- The UK Faculty of Public Health is a professional body for professionals with an interest in population health: www.fph.org.uk.

- The Health and Safety Executive has information about occupational health: www.hse.gov.uk.

- The Health Protection Agency is an NHS body responsible for public health in England: www.hpa.org.uk.

The ten Wilson and Junger[29] criteria for a screening programme

- Is the disease an important public health problem?

- Is there an effective treatment for localised disease?

- Are facilities for further diagnosis and treatment available?

- Is there an identifiable latent or early symptomatic stage of disease?

- Is the technique to be used for screening effective?

- Are the tests acceptable to the population?

- Is the natural history of the disease known?

- Is there a strategy for determining which patients should and should not be treated?

- Is the cost of screening acceptable?

- Is effective treatment available and does management of cases in the early stages have a favourable impact on prognosis?

Statement 3.02: *Genetics in Primary Care*

Genetics is a rapidly evolving area of medicine that, in particular, requires GPs to keep their skills and knowledge up to date. About one in ten patients seen in primary care has a disorder with a genetic component. GPs must identify patients and families who have, or are at risk of, genetic conditions, sensitively communicate genetic information, and provide tailored support and advice.

Taking and interpreting a family history is particularly important for identifying those at risk of common conditions such as cancer, cardiovascular disease and diabetes, as well as Mendelian genetic disorders. GPs must also be able to advise patients about the genetic aspects of antenatal and newborn screening. GPs play a key role in identifying patients and families who would benefit from referral to specialist genetic services and, as genetic conditions are often multi-systemic, in coordinating patient care with other services.

The condensed knowledge

		☑ or score (1–5)
Symptoms	Symptoms and signs of genetic conditions vary widely, particularly in autosomal dominant conditions where symptoms may vary in number and severity between affected patients within the same family (e.g. variability of expression in neurofibromatosis). It is important for GPs to become familiar with the common autosomal dominant and recessive conditions (see below)	
	Anxiety about a family history of a disease, for example if a relative has been recently diagnosed with cancer, is also a common presentation	
Conditions	Examples of common chromosome anomalies:	
	• Down's syndrome	
	• Turner syndrome	
	• Klinefelter's syndrome	
	• translocations	

		☑ **or score** **(1–5)**
Conditions	Autosomal dominant disorders:	
	• familial hypercholesterolaemia	
	• adult polycystic kidney disease	_____
	• neurofibromatosis	_____
	• Huntington's disease	_____
	• hypercholesterolaemia	_____
	Recessive single-gene disorders:	
	• cystic fibrosis	
	• haemoglobinopathies (sickle-cell disease, thalassaemias)	_____
	• haemochromatosis	_____
	X-linked single-gene disorders:	
	• Duchenne and Becker muscular dystrophies	
	• haemophilia A	_____
	• fragile X	_____
	Disorders with a genetic component (e.g. bipolar disorder, cerebrovascular disease, cardiovascular disease, Alzheimer's, asthma)	
	Common familial cancers (e.g. breast, colon)	_____
	Conditions exhibiting variable inheritance patterns (e.g. inherited forms of deafness, muscular dystrophies)	_____
Investigation	Knowledge of principles of genetic tests: diagnostic, predictive, carrier status	
Treatment	Varies depending on the individual disease but includes, for example, regular surveillance or family-planning options	

Continued over

	☑ or score (1–5)
Prevention	The preventive measures and surveillance options available for those at risk of developing some genetic conditions, for example:
	• direct surveillance (e.g. regular colonoscopy)
	• early treatment (e.g. statins for hypercholesterolaemia)
	• lifestyle advice (e.g. smoking cessation in alpha 1-antitrypsin deficiency)
	• preventive surgery (e.g. mastectomy, oophorectomy)
	• imaging (e.g. adult polycystic kidney disease, breast cancer)
	• newborn screening programme for phenylketonuria (PKU)
	Tip: See www.newbornbloodspot.screening.nhs.uk

The condensed skills

	☑ or score (1–5)
Communication skills	Conveying information about genetics in an understandable way; helping patients make informed decisions, bearing in mind the issues around confidentiality when other family members may be affected
Consultation skills	Discussing genetic conditions in a non-directive and non-judgemental manner:
	being aware that people have different attitudes and beliefs about inheritance
	ensuring your own beliefs do not influence the content of the consultation and the management options offered to a patient

	☑ or score (1–5)
Cognitive skills Taking and interpreting a family history (or 'pedigree') to identify patients with, or at risk of, a genetic condition.	
Tip: *The e-GP 'Genetics in primary care' course has e-learning sessions on how to draw and interpret a family pedigree (www.e-GP.org)*	
How to use online risk assessment tools	

The condensed know-how

	☑ or score (1–5)
Patterns of inheritance: single gene (e.g. autosomal dominant, recessive, X-linked), chromosomal, mitochondrial and multifactorial	
The heterogeneity in genetic diseases and understanding the principles of assessing genetic risk, including the principles of: • risk estimates for family members of patients with Mendelian diseases • recurrence risk for simple chromosome anomalies, e.g. trisomies	
The organisation of genetics services, where to obtain specialist help and how to make appropriate referrals to genetics services. **Tip:** *There is a national database of genetic centres on the British Society for Human Genetics website: www.bshg.org.uk*	
The support services available for those with a genetic condition. **Tip:** *Contact a Family offers information on genetic disorders and enables families affected by rare conditions to get in touch with other affected families: www.cafamily.org.uk*	
The different uses of genetic tests (diagnostic, predictive, carrier testing) and their limitations. **Tip:** *Information on genetic testing can be found at: www.ukgtn.nhs.uk*	

Continued over

	☑ **or score** **(1–5)**
The genetic aspects of antenatal and newborn screening programmes (e.g. Down's syndrome, sickle-cell and thalassaemia), and their indications, uses and limitations. **Tip:** *Useful information on the NHS antenatal and newborn screening programmes is available at: www.screening.nhs.uk*	_____
Systems for following up patients who have, or are at risk of, a genetic condition and have chosen to undergo regular surveillance. **Tip:** *Does your practice records system have a diary or reminder function?*	_____
The reproductive options available to those with a known genetic condition (e.g. adoption; gamete donation and prenatal diagnosis)	_____
How the make-up of the local population may affect the prevalence of genetic conditions and attitudes towards genetic disease	_____
How a patient's cultural and religious background and beliefs concerning inheritance are important when providing care for people with, or at risk of, genetic conditions. **Tip:** *For example, some patients mistakenly assume that their genetic risk is related to the degree of resemblance to the affected family member*	_____
The social and psychological impacts of a genetic condition on the patient and his or her family, dependants and employment	_____
Awareness that it is not always possible to determine the cause of a condition that may be genetic or the mutation responsible (e.g. intellectual disability)	_____
Local and national referral guidelines for patients with a family history of a condition that may require genetic investigations or screening (e.g. breast, colon cancer)	_____
Local and national referral guidelines for managing patients with identified genetic conditions (e.g. familial hypercholesterolaemia, sickle-cell). **Tip:** *NICE guidance on* Identification and Management of Familial Hypercholesterolaemia *is available at: www.nice.org.uk/CG071*	_____

	☑ **or score**
	(1–5)

The ethical, legal and social implications of genetic information and how it impacts not only on the patient but also on the family, and awareness that a genetic diagnosis in an individual may have wide-ranging implications for children and other family members.

Tip: *Consider the possible implications of genetic testing on children or on the ability to obtain certain types of insurance*

Issues of confidentiality arising when information about one individual can be used in a predictive manner for another family member.

Tip: *The GMC guidance* Confidentiality *(2009) is available on the GMC website at: www.gmc-uk.org/guidance/ethical_guidance/confidentiality.asp*

The condensed resources

- NICE clinical guidelines relevant to this section include *Familial Breast Cancer* and *Familial Hypercholesterolaemia*. Available at: http://guidance.nice.org.uk/CG/Published.

- *e*-GP contains RCGP e-learning sessions on taking, drawing and interpreting genetic family histories, communicating genetic information and managing patients: www.e-GP.org.

- British Society for Human Genetics has a directory of UK genetics centres: www.bshg.org.uk.

- The NHS National Genetics Education and Development Centre provides education and training in genetics and resources to help with taking a family history: www.geneticseducation.nhs.uk.

- The Primary Care Genetics Society website contains information resources on the management of genetic conditions in primary care: www.pcgs.org.uk.

- Unique provides information and support on rare chromosomal disorders: www.rarechromo.org.

Statement 3.03: *Care of Acutely Ill People*

Acutely ill people of all ages present unpredictably in general practice and require an urgent response, sometimes interrupting normal work routines. The effective management of an acutely ill person includes competent recognition, assessment and immediate management. Organisation, teamwork, communication and situational awareness are also important aspects. A GP must make patient safety a priority and consider the appropriateness of interventions according to a patient's wishes, the severity of the illness and any chronic or co-morbid diseases. GPs must accept responsibility for taking action, at the same time recognising a need to involve more experienced personnel when appropriate, and must keep their resuscitation skills up to date.

Urgent care includes both in-hours and out-of-hours emergencies but particular features of working out of hours, such as isolation, the relative lack of supporting services and the need to support self-care, require a specific educational focus.

The condensed knowledge

		☑ or score (1–5)
Symptoms	Cardiovascular – chest pain, haemorrhage, shock	
	Respiratory – wheeze, breathlessness, stridor, choking	
	Central nervous system – convulsions, reduced conscious level, confusion, unconsciousness	
	Collapse	
	Mental health – threatened self-harm, delusional states, violent patients	
	Severe pain	
Conditions	Acute coronary syndromes	
	Anaphylaxis	
	Appendicitis	
	Arrhythmias	
	Asthma	

		☑ **or score** **(1–5)**
Conditions	Bowel obstruction and perforation	
	Common problems that may be expected with certain practice activities: anaphylaxis after immunisation, local anaesthetic toxicity and vaso-vagal attacks (e.g. during minor surgery or IUD insertion)	
	Dissecting aneurysms	
	Ectopic pregnancy and antenatal emergencies	
	Haemorrhage (revealed or concealed)	
	Ischaemia	
	Loss of consciousness	
	Malignant hypertension	
	Meningitis and septicaemia	
	Parasuicide and suicide attempts	
	Pulmonary embolus	
	Pulmonary oedema (severe)	
	Shock (including no cardiac output)	
	Status epilepticus	
	Understand the principles of managing dangerous diagnoses.	
	Tip: *See 'Dangerous diagnoses' box on p. 186*	
Investigation	Blood glucose	
	Performing and interpreting an ECG	
	Other investigations are rare in primary care because acutely ill patients needing investigation are usually referred to secondary care	
Resources	Appropriate use of emergency services, including logistics of how to obtain an ambulance/paramedic crew	

Continued over

	☑ or score (1–5)
Resources — Familiarity with available equipment in own bag / car / practice and that carried by emergency services. **Tip:** *This information should be provided in an induction programme – if not, find out where the emergency equipment is kept and how to use it before an emergency occurs!*	
Selection and maintenance of the appropriate equipment and un-expired drugs that should be carried by GPs. **Tip:** *There is a useful summary of what to put in a doctor's bag on Patient.co.uk at: www.patient.co.uk/ doctor/The-Doctor%27s-Bag-Contents.htm*	
Being able to organise and lead a response when required, which may include participation by staff, members of the public or qualified responders	
Knowledge of training required for practice staff and others (as a team) in the appropriate responses to an acutely ill person	
Prevention — Advice to patients on prevention, e.g. with a patient with known heart disease this includes advice on how to manage ischaemic pain, including use of glyceryl trinitrate (GTN), aspirin and appropriate first-line use of paramedic ambulance	

The condensed skills

	☑ or score (1–5)
Communication skills — Dealing sensitively with people who may have a serious diagnosis (including those who refuse admission) and presenting a balanced view of the benefits and harms of medical treatment, while being aware how acute illness itself and the anxiety caused by it can impair communication	

		☑ **or score (1–5)**
Consultation skills	Skills to consult safely and effectively on the telephone with people who may be acutely ill; evaluating patient risk, giving advice and making appropriate arrangements to see the patient	
	The appropriate use of open and closed questions to gather specific information in an urgent situation	
	Arranging further monitoring and review of acutely ill patients as required to reassess their condition and determine changes to the initial management plan	
	Safety-netting skills to inform patients of the expected progression of their condition, indications that mean further review is needed, and how to access further advice	
Decision-making skills	Assessing and managing common medical, surgical and psychiatric emergencies in the in-hours and out-of-hours settings, often without access to previous records	
	Deciding whether to admit, refer or seek advice about an acutely ill person and not being unduly influenced by others (such as professional colleagues who have not assessed the patient).	
	Tip: *Emergency situations sometimes require more directive approaches to team leadership (e.g. running a resuscitation)*	
Procedures	● Performing and interpreting an ECG	
	● The 'ABC' principles, basic life support of children and adults, and use of an automated defibrillator	
	● Controlling a haemorrhage	
	● Immediate management of anaphylaxis	
	● Suturing a wound	
	● Using a nebuliser	

Continued over

		☑ **or score** **(1–5)**
Risk management skills	Managing personal security and risks to yourself, the patient and others	
Housekeeping skills	Coping with the emotional and stressful aspects of providing acute care	

The condensed know-how

	☑ **or score** **(1–5)**
How to recognise, evaluate and manage acutely ill patients, including knowledge of the key differential diagnoses for acutely presenting symptoms. **Tip:** *GPs are unlikely to see acutely ill patients with rare conditions very often. Consider keeping easy-to-access protocols in your doctor's bag. Review the Acute Competencies from Foundation Years 1 and 2*	
Know the symptoms and signs of severe illnesses that may be diagnostically overshadowed by less severe illnesses and have strategies to avoid this (e.g. the finding of otitis media in a child does not negate the need to assess for possible meningococcal infection)	
Protecting patients with non-urgent and self-limiting problems from being over-investigated, over-treated or deprived of their liberty	
How age, gender, ethnicity, pregnancy, treatment, chronic or co-morbid disease and previous health factors may affect the risk and presentation of acute illness (e.g. in the very old or young). **Tip:** *Always consider ectopic pregnancy as a possible cause of abdominal or pelvic pain in a woman of fertile age*	
The response time required in order to optimise the outcome for the patient (e.g. 'the golden hour')	
An understanding of local and national protocols, and sources of evidence relating to emergency care and how these may be adapted to unusual circumstances. **Tip:** *Resuscitation and other emergency protocols are available from the UK Resuscitation Council (www.resus.org.uk)*	

	☑ **or score** **(1–5)**
Methods for transporting patients to secondary care and factors to consider when deciding the chosen method and urgency, including when to call 999	
Factors affecting continuity of care in acute illness and steps for minimising problems, including handover and follow-up arrangements.	
Tip: *Review the quality of the A&E discharge summaries received by your practice and the issues this raises*	
Factors for deciding in whom resuscitation or intensive care might be inappropriate and how to seek advice on this from carers and colleagues.	
Tip: *The Resuscitation Council (www.resus.org.uk) publishes a guideline on 'Do Not Resuscitate' order*	
How to recognise, confirm, record and certify death, the role of the coroner (or procurator fiscal) and how to provide immediate bereavement support and your obligations when dealing with an expected or an unexpected death.	
Tip: *Make sure you know what to do if you are called to certify a death at home. This includes providing relevant practical information for the family*	
The needs of carers and family at the time of the acutely ill person's presentation and conflicts regarding management that may exist between patients and their relatives.	
Tip: *Consider in which limited situations patient autonomy can be overruled (e.g. mental health emergencies)*	
How the presentation of patients with chronic conditions to urgent care services is influenced by their management in primary care	
Ways of recognising and managing patients who are likely to need acute care in the future, and ways to offer them advice on prevention, effective self-management and when and who to call for help.	
Tip: *Find out about case management of those at high risk of admission*	
Local specialist community resources for acute care or less acute assessment or rehabilitation and how to use these resources appropriately	
The impact of the doctor's working environment and resources on how acute care is provided.	
Tip: *Make sure you know where your practice keeps emergency equipment and who is responsible for its maintenance and upkeep*	

Continued over

	☑ **or score****(1–5)**

The need for leadership, a team approach and an understanding of the roles of the practice staff in responding to requests for help and managing acutely ill patients and their relatives.

Tip: *Do you have a practice protocol in place for dealing with a major incident or flu pandemic?*

How national NHS emergency and out-of-hours care is organised, and the local arrangements for the provision of out-of-hours care

Understanding of the out-of-hours organisation(s) in which you work, including:

- IT and communication systems

- how to record and transmit information about patients and the outcomes of contact (to preserve continuity of care)

- how to organise working sessions or shifts

- the reporting of significant events and near misses

Cultural and other individual factors that might affect emergency management of patients.

Does the patient have specific cultural or religious beliefs that you should take into account (e.g. Jehovah's Witness) or a living will?

Legal frameworks affecting acute healthcare provision, especially regarding compulsory admission and treatment.

Tip: *Familiarise yourself with the key sections of the Mental Health Act*

Patient rights to autonomy and factors that affect an acutely ill patient's capacity for autonomy and the need to respect advanced care planning decisions.

Tip: *Read up about capacity to consent and the Mental Capacity Act 2005*

The condensed resources

- NICE clinical guidelines relevant to this section include *Anaphylaxis, Bacterial Meningitis and Meningococcal Septicaemia, Chest Pain of Recent Onset* and *Stroke*. Available at: http://guidance.nice.org.uk/CG/Published.

- SIGN guidelines relevant to this section includes *Acute Coronary Syndromes, British Guideline on the Management of Asthma* (joint with British Thoracic Society, quick reference guide in the BNF), *Early Management of Patients with a Head Injury, Management of Invasive Meningococcal Disease in Children and Young People* and *Management of Patients with Stroke or TIA*. Available at: www.sign.ac.uk/guidelines.

- UK resuscitation guidelines can be found on the UK Resuscitation Council website, as well as guidelines on managing anaphylaxis and other emergencies in the community: www.resus.org.uk.

- COGPED has produced a position paper that sets out the standards for out-of-hours GP training (available on their website at: www.cogped.org.uk/page.php?id=199).

- The RCGP report *Guidance for Commissioning Integrated Urgent and Emergency Care: a 'whole system' approach* is available on the RCGP website at: www.rcgp.org.uk/centre_for_commissioning/publications_and_resources.aspx.

- *e*-GP contains RCGP e-learning sessions on basic life support, managing major incidents, burns and scalds, and limb and head injuries.

- Doctors.net (www.doctors.net.uk) contains learning modules on various aspects of emergency care.

- GPnotebook (www.gpnotebook.co.uk) contains clinical information on managing acute medical conditions.

Dangerous diagnoses

Research carried out by the Medical Protection Society[32] has identified a number of diagnoses that demand urgent action when the suspicion of them crosses a doctor's mind. Adverse events occur more frequently when a doctor has suspected a potentially dangerous diagnosis but not acted to rule out this possibility. Dangerous diagnoses include:

- myocardial infarction
- pulmonary embolus
- subarachnoid haemorrhage
- appendicitis
- limb ischaemia
- intestinal obstruction or perforation
- meningitis
- aneurysms
- ectopic pregnancy
- acute psychosis/mania
- visual problems that could lead to blindness including retinal detachment and haemorrhage as well as systemic disease such as temporal arteritis.

As a general rule, if a GP suspects a dangerous diagnosis is possible, he or she should act as if the diagnosis was certain and refer the patient to the nearest emergency centre. The GP may well be wrong but without having access to appropriate investigations it is far better to be safe than sorry.

Statement 3.04: *Care of Children and Young People*

Most care for children and young people occurs in the community and there is evidence that good primary care delivers improved health outcomes. A child's experiences in early life have a crucial impact on his or her life chances. Promoting health can be included in all contacts with a child or young person and his or her family; this should be targeted particularly at those who are vulnerable or socially excluded.

Safeguarding children and young people requires all GPs to be effective at recognising and dealing with child abuse and neglect. GPs should respond to the needs of children and young people in special circumstances, through referral and joint working with relevant services, and should be aware that the needs of young people are different from those of younger children, particularly in terms of their health problems, consent, confidentiality and communication issues.

The condensed knowledge

		☑ **or score** **(1–5)**
Symptoms	Abdominal pain (acute and chronic)	
	Behavioural problems	
	Developmental delay	
	Failure to thrive and growth disorders	
	Vomiting, fever, drowsiness	
	Early presenting symptoms and signs of cancers (e.g. brain tumours, leukaemia, retinoblastoma, sarcoma)	
Conditions	Bronchiolitis	
	Child abuse, non-accidental injury and neglect	
	Chronic disease in children: asthma, diabetes, arthritis, intellectual disability (see other statements)	
	Constipation	
	Cough/dyspnoea, wheezing including respiratory infections	

Continued over

		☑ **or score** **(1–5)**
Conditions	Developmental problems (e.g. autistic spectrum disorder and related conditions)	
	Epilepsy	
	Foreign bodies (e.g. nose, ears, swallowing, inhaling)	
	Gastroenteritis	
	Infant colic	
	Meningitis	
	Mental health problems such as attention deficit hyperactivity disorder, depression, eating disorders, substance misuse and self-harm	
	Neonatal problems:	
	• birthmarks	
	• early feeding problems	
	• heart murmur	
	• jaundice	
	• poor weight gain	
	• sticky eye	
	Normal development and developmental problems (physical and psychological)	
	Otitis media	
	Psychological problems: enuresis, encopresis, bullying, school refusal, behaviour disorders including tantrums	
	Pyrexia and febrile convulsions	
	Sensory deficit (e.g. hearing or visual impairment)	
	Sudden Infant Death Syndrome (SIDS) and strategies to reduce risk	
	Urinary tract infection	
	Viral exanthems (childhood illnesses associated with rashes)	

		☑ or score (1–5)
Prevention	Alcohol and drug screening and interventions	
	Breastfeeding	
	Healthy diet and exercise for children and young people	
	Immunisation programmes for children	
	Keeping children and young people safe: child protection, accident prevention	
	Prenatal diagnosis	
	Reducing the risk of teenagers getting pregnant or acquiring sexually transmitted infections	
	Smoking cessation	
	Social and emotional wellbeing	

The condensed skills

		☑ or score (1–5)
Communication skills	Listening and responding to the sensitivities, health attitudes and behaviours of children and young people, and communicating with parents, carers and families	
Consultation skills	Enabling children and young people to participate in informed decisions about their care, taking into account their age and development	
	Consultation skills for younger children	
	Skills to encourage and support parents in self-care	
Examination skills	The examination of the newborn child	
	The six-week check	

Continued over

The condensed know-how

	☑ or score (1–5)
Safe prescribing in children and young people:	
● calculating drug doses for infants and children	
● the indications, contraindications, risks and benefits of medicines in children and young people.	
Tip: *The BNF for children is a great resource for paediatric prescribing: www.bnfc.org*	
Information to enable parents or carers, children and young people to manage minor illnesses themselves, to use community pharmacists and triage services, and to access appropriate medical services when necessary. **Tip:** *Patients can obtain free advice on managing minor illness from NHS Direct: www.nhsdirect.nhs.uk*	
Issues around parents with special needs, the role of fathers in parenting, and how to support children of parents with substance misuse, mental health problems or chronic illnesses	
How to promote physical health, mental health and emotional wellbeing, and encourage children, young people and their families to develop healthy lifestyles	
National immunisation programmes and the GP's role in promoting and organising immunisation. **Tip:** *This information is contained in the DH's Green Book* (Immunisation against Infectious Disease). *This can be found at: www.immunisation. dh.gov.uk/category/the-green-book*	
The GP's role in the prevention of accidents. **Tip:** *You can find more information on promoting safety from the Royal Society for the Prevention of Accidents (www.rospa.com)*	
Common neonatal problems including feeding problems, colic, breastfeeding and nutrition	

	☑ **or score**
	(1–5)

Normal growth and development of children and young people, and management of delayed development and failure to thrive.

Tip: *Familiarise yourself with the use of growth centile charts and common developmental milestones. Centile charts are available on the Royal College of Paediatrics and Child Health website at: www.rcpch.ac.uk/growthcharts*

Problems during transition from child to adolescent, and adolescent to adult, and the effects on the vulnerable or those with chronic diseases.

Tip: *Find out about children's and young people's experiences of ill health at: www.youthhealthtalk.org*

How to recognise children and young people at risk, identify vulnerability factors for children and young people in special circumstances, and make appropriate referral.

Tip: *All healthcare professionals are required to obtain a Criminal Records Bureau disclosure and to regularly undertake training in child safeguarding*

The significance of non-attendance:

- can be an indicator of a family's vulnerability, potentially placing the child's welfare in jeopardy

- can also be an indicator that services are difficult for families and young people to access or considered inappropriate, and need reviewing

- (in primary or secondary care) should be followed up – remember that a child is reliant on a carer to take them.

Tip: *Does your practice have a policy for managing 'DNA's?*

Coordinating care for children and families, acting as an advocate when required, and recognising and managing issues around multi-agency working (working across professional and agency boundaries).

Tip: *Familiarise yourself with the safeguarding issues arising from the tragic cases of Victoria Climbié and Baby Peter*

Continued over

	☑ **or score**
	(1–5)

Understand the GP's key role in the safeguarding of children and young people, recognising that:

- the welfare of the child is paramount

- attention on the family may risk losing sight of the child, especially if the parents have challenging problems of their own

- the clinical features of child abuse, neglect and non-accidental injury, knowing about local arrangements for child protection, referring effectively and playing a part in assessment and continuing management (including prevention).

Tip: *Familiarise yourself with your local child safeguarding arrangements and the contact details of your safeguarding lead. If possible try to attend a child protection case conference meeting*

Improving welfare of the unborn baby and reducing the impact of parental problems including domestic violence, substance misuse and mental health problems, how to recognise such problems (and make a sensitive enquiry) and how to access the relevant local services

Family, socioeconomic and environmental factors, including school, community, ethnicity, cultural issues, inequalities and parenting capacity, that affect health and wellbeing in children and young people, and vulnerability factors for children in special circumstances

Issues around design and delivery of services for young people, relating to access, communication, confidentiality and consent.

Tip: *The GMC has produced* 0-18 Years: guidance for all doctors *(2007), which is available on its website at: www.gmc-uk.org/guidance/ethi-cal_guidance/children_guidance_index.asp*

Issues around access for young people to confidential contraceptive and sexual health advice, the design of services tailored to meet their specific needs and the relevant updated guidance.

Tip: *Familiarise yourself with the principles of Gillick/Fraser competence and the best-practice guidance issued by the DH* [33]

The role of the health visitor and how to undertake a comprehensive child and family needs assessment.

Tip: *Spend a day with a health visitor – health visitors know lots of practical tips and advice on everyday child-rearing and behavioural problems*

	☑ **or score (1–5)**
The legal and political context and the organisation of child and adolescent care in the NHS, including care pathways and local systems of care	
The impact of disability on the child or young person and his or her family. **Tip:** *Do a case study centred on a child registered at your practice with disability*	
The impact of inequalities on children and their families, and steps to address these	
Recognising inappropriate eating habits such as anorexia nervosa or bulimia and appropriate interventions and services. **Tip:** *NICE has published guidelines on eating disorders (www.nice.org.uk)*	
The issues around treating children and young people equitably and with respect for their beliefs, preferences, dignity and rights (and the relevant legislation), and the issues around confidentiality and consent, record-keeping and sharing information (including legal aspects) relevant to minors	

The condensed resources

- NICE clinical guidelines relevant to this section include *Atopic Eczema in Children, Attention Deficit Hyperactivity Disorder, Autism in Children and Young People, Constipation in Children and Young People, Depression in Children and Young People, Diarrhoea and Vomiting in Children under 5, Feverish Illness in Children, Food Allergy in Children and Young People, Nocturnal Enuresis, Urinary Tract Infection in Children* and *When to Suspect Child Maltreatment*. Available at: http://guidance.nice.org.uk/CG/Published.

- SIGN guidelines relevant to this section include *Management of Attention Deficit and Hyperkinetic Disorders in Children and Young People, Assessment, Diagnosis and Clinical Interventions for Children and Young People with Autistic Spectrum Disorders, Bronchiolitis in Children, Diagnosis and Management of Epilepsies in Children* and *Diagnosis and Management of Childhood Otitis Media in Primary Care*. Available at: www.sign.ac.uk/guidelines.

- BNF for Children contains specific information on prescribing in children: www.bnfc.org.

- *e*-GP contains RCGP e-learning sessions on the care of neonates and infants, care of children, adolescent health, health promotion and safeguarding children: www.e-GP.org.

- The Great Ormond Street website has information for professionals and parents: www.gosh.nhs.uk.

- Teenage-friendly health advice: www.teenagehealthfreak.org.

- The Royal College of Psychiatrists produces a popular series of leaflets on mental health and behavioural problems in children called *Mental Health and Growing Up*, available at: www.rcpsych.ac.uk.

- The RCGP and Royal College of Nursing (RCN) joint publication *Getting it Right for Teenagers in Your Practice* (2002) is available on the RCN website at: www.rcn.org.uk/members/downloads/getting_it_right.pdf.

- The DH's *Healthy Child Programme: pregnancy and the first five years of life* is available on the DH's website at: www.dh.gov.uk/en/Publicationsandstatistics/Publications/PublicationsPolicyAndGuidance/DH_107563.

- A summary of the national strategy for child health in England is available at: www.nhs.uk/NHSEngland/NSF/Pages/Children.aspx.

Statement 3.05: *Care of Older Adults*

The UK has an ageing population and the care of older people forms a significant part of everyday general practice. Key issues in the care of older people include multiple co-morbidity, difficulties in communicating, loss of autonomy, the problems of polypharmacy and the need for additional support. GPs have an essential role to play in supporting older people and their carers, in partnership with the wider health and social care team, in the consulting room, the patient's own home, and in the local community.

The condensed skills

		☑ or score (1–5)
Clinical management skills	Managing the concurrent health problems experienced by older people through identification, exploration, negotiation, acceptance and prioritisation	
Communication skills	Recognising the challenges of communicating with older patients including the slower tempo, possible unreliability of the history and the evidence of third parties	
	Ability to engage, agree and coordinate care with carers, family members and other team members as appropriate	
Consultation skills	Developing and maintaining a relationship style that treats the older patient with respect and does not patronise	
Mental health assessment skills	Assessing brain function and mood (e.g. using short mental state questionnaires), and evaluating the testimony of third parties	

The condensed know-how

	☑ or score (1–5)
The epidemiology of older people's problems in primary care in the context of knowledge of the practice community (e.g. number of elderly patients, prevalence of chronic diseases)	
How the pattern of alarm symptoms and signs suggestive of serious disease (e.g. malignancy) may present differently in older adults and how to recognise and respond to suspected cancer early and appropriately	
The theories of ageing; the physical (including lab values), psychological and social changes that occur with age and relating them to the adaptations that an older person makes to compensate (and the eventual breakdown of these adaptations)	
The effect of physical factors, particularly diet, exercise, temperature and sleep, on the health of older people and the inter-relationships between health and social care	
The concept of co-morbidity and the central role of the GP in providing coordinated and comprehensive care for people with multiple conditions, and for ensuring integrated care for patients with multiple and complex conditions	
Features relating to prognosis of diseases in old age and how this informs an appropriate plan for further investigation and management	
The management of the conditions and problems commonly associated with old age, such as Parkinson's disease, falls, gait disorders, stroke, cancers, dementia, depression, anxiety and confusion. **Tip:** *The Royal College of Physicians (RCP) produces guidance in this area, available at: www.rcplondon.ac.uk/specialty/geriatric-medicine*	
Drug treatment in the elderly, the physiology of absorption, metabolism and excretion of drugs, the hazards posed by multiple prescribing, non-compliance and iatrogenic disease, the importance of medication reviews and the issue of medication errors and iatrogenic disease. **Tip:** *Review the concept of polypharmacy and the Beers criteria [34] (medication inappropriate for elderly people); the BNF has a section on prescribing in the elderly*	

	☑ **or score**
	(1–5)

Issues around access to care for older people, including geographical distance, appropriate timing of appointments and the organisational approach to the management of chronic conditions and co-morbidities	

Knowledge of the locally agreed protocols for preventing and managing health problems in the elderly (e.g. transient ischaemic attack [TIA], falls, memory problems). **Tip:** *Consider spending time with a local geriatrician and find out what specialist services are available in your area. Do you have a local geriatric day hospital? A rapid access clinic? A falls clinic? A TIA clinic?*	

Issues around the transfer from one system of care to another, the complications that can arise and how they can be prevented and managed. **Tip:** *Consider spending time with a local geriatrician and find out what specialist services are available in your area. Do you have a local geriatric day hospital?*	

Support services for older patients and their carers (e.g. podiatry, visual and hearing aids, immobility and walking aids, meals on wheels, home care services), different forms of day care and residential accommodation, and the various statutory and voluntary organisations for older people in the community. **Tip:** *District nurses are often excellent sources of this information*	

Organisational aspects of care for older people and their carers in the practice, including appointment systems, carers' support programmes, policies on repeat prescriptions, the appropriate use of screening and case-finding programmes, and auditing the quality of care. **Tip:** *Review your practice's repeat prescribing policy and the procedure for medication reviews and carer health checks*	

How the provision of care can affect the patient's sense of identity and dignity, and ways of ensuring patients are not discriminated against due to their age, and how to recognise and respond to elder abuse	

The special features of mental health problems in old age, the features of dementia, and the effects of physical function on the mental state. **Tip:** *See the RCGP online course 'Mental health in older people' (www.elearning.rcgp.org.uk)*	

Continued over

	☑ **or score (1–5)**
Ethical and cultural tensions between the needs of the elderly individual and the community. **Tip:** *Consider the ethical problems raised when advising an elderly patient on his or her fitness to drive and the Driver and Vehicle Licensing Agency (DVLA) regulations*	
How preventive strategies can be adapted to older people and the steps that can be taken to reduce inequalities in healthcare provision. **Tip:** *Look into strategies for preventing falls in the elderly*	
The legal issues relevant to the elderly including confidentiality, Mental Health Act, power of attorney, court of protection, guardianship, living wills, death certification and cremation. **Tip:** *Have a tutorial on the paperwork related to death, in particular when it is necessary to involve the police or the coroner.* **Tip:** *The forms for power of attorney (in England) can be found at: www.justice.gov.uk/about/opg*	
The key government policy documents, national guidelines and research findings that influence healthcare provision for older people. **Tip:** *The Scottish* Adding Life to Years *(Report of the Expert Group on Healthcare of Older People)*[35] *is available on the Scottish government website at: www.scotland.gov.uk/Publications/2002/01/10624/File-1*	

The condensed resources

- NICE clinical guidelines relevant to this section include *Delirium, Dementia and Falls*. Others are listed in the specific clinical examples (particularly 3.12 *Cardiovascular Health* and 3.18 *Care of People with Neurological Problems*). Available at: http://guidance.nice.org.uk/CG/Published.

- The NICE dementia quality standard is available at: www.nice.org.uk/guidance/qualitystandards/dementia/dementiaqualitystandard.jsp.

- SIGN guidelines relevant to this section include *Management of Patients with Dementia*. Available at: www.sign.ac.uk/guidelines.

- *e*-GP contains RCGP e-learning sessions on a range of topics relevant to the care of older adults (www.e-GP.org).

- The NSF for older people is available on the DH website at: www.dh.gov.uk/en/Publicationsandstatistics/Publications/PublicationsPolicyAndGuidance/DH_4003066. A summary can be found at: www.nhs.uk/NHSEngland/NSF/Pages/Olderpeople.aspx.

- The DVLA guidelines can be found at: www.dft.gov.uk/dvla/medical/ataglance.aspx.

- Age UK offers information and support for the elderly on health and social care: www.ageuk.org.uk.

- The British Geriatrics Society is the professional body for specialists in old-age medicine and psychiatry of old age: www.bgs.org.uk.

Statement 3.06: *Women's Health*

Women's health matters, including contraception, pregnancy, menopause and disorders of the reproductive organs, account for around a quarter of general practice workload. In society, women generally tend to play a larger role in caring for dependent relatives and children, and GPs play an important part in supporting women in this role and in organising women-friendly services. GPs are also responsible for diagnosing domestic violence and dealing with its physical and psychological effects.

The condensed knowledge

		☑ **or score (1–5)**
Symptoms	Breast pain, breast lumps, distortion, nipple discharge	
	Dyspareunia	
	Emotional problems, including low mood and symptoms of depression	
	Faecal incontinence	
	Infertility – primary and secondary	
	Menopause and menopausal problems	
	Pelvic pain	
	Period-related problems	
	Post-menopausal bleeding	
	Pruritus vulvae and vaginal discharge	
	Urinary malfunction: dysuria, frequency, incontinence	
Conditions	Female-specific conditions, including:	
	• abnormal cervical cytology	
	• benign breast conditions	
	• breast cancer	

		☑ **or score** **(1–5)**
Conditions	• gynaecological infections, including Bartholin's abscess	_____
	• gynaecological malignancies (e.g. ovarian, endometrial, cervical)	_____
	• pelvic inflammatory disease	_____
	• uterine conditions (e.g. fibroids, polyps)	_____
	• vaginal and uterine prolapse	_____
	Menstrual disorders:	
	• amenorrhoea	_____
	• dysmenorrhoea	_____
	• inter-menstrual bleeding	_____
	• irregular bleeding patterns	_____
	• menorrhagia	_____
	• pre-menstrual syndrome	
	Mental health issues more prevalent in women, including anxiety, depression, parasuicide, eating disorders and self-harming (and the relationship between these, adolescence, pregnancy and the menopause)	_____
	Pregnancy-related problems (as well as normal antenatal and postnatal care):	
	Tip: *Spend a day on attachment with the community midwife*	_____
	• abnormal lies and placenta praevia	_____
	• anaemia	_____
	• antepartum haemorrhage, abruption, post-partum haemorrhage	_____

Continued over

	☑ **or score (1–5)**
Conditions	

- constipation and haemorrhoids
- deep-vein thrombosis and pulmonary embolism, post-dates, reduced movements
- ectopic pregnancy
- hyperemesis
- gastro-oesophageal reflux disease (GORD)
- gestational diabetes
- intrauterine death
- miscarriage and abortion
- multiple pregnancy
- musculoskeletal problems (e.g. back pain, symphysis pubis dysfunction, leg ache and varicose veins)
- obstetric complications requiring specialist monitoring (e.g. poly- and oligohydramnios, growth retardation and foetal abnormality)
- pre-eclampsia and hypertension in pregnancy
- post-dates or reduced movements
- premature labour
- rhesus status and role of anti-D
- trophoblastic disease
- venous thrombo-embolism in pregnancy

Sexual dysfunction including psychosexual conditions

		☑ **or score** (1–5)
Investigation	Pregnancy testing	
	Urinalysis, mid-stream specimen of urine (MSU) and urine dipstick	
	Blood tests including renal function tests, hormone tests	
	Bacteriological and virology tests	
	Knowledge of secondary care investigations including colposcopy and fertility investigations	
Treatment	Primary care management of the conditions listed above	
	Menopause management including the pros and cons of hormone replacement therapy (HRT)	
	Knowledge of specialist treatments and surgical procedures including: laparoscopy, dilatation and curettage (D&C), hysterectomy, oophorectomy, ovarian cystectomy, pelvic floor repair, medical and surgical termination of pregnancy, sterilisation	
	Understand the risks of prescribing during pregnancy	
Prevention	Breast cancer screening	
	Cervical cancer screening and human papilloma virus (HPV) triage	
	HPV vaccination programme	
	Pre-pregnancy issues including folic acid, vitamin D, family and genetic history, diet and lifestyle advice	
	Pregnancy care including health promotion, antenatal screening and diagnosis, social and cultural factors, smoking and alcohol, diet, age factors and previous obstetric history	
	Rubella testing and immunisation	
	Risk assessment, screening and management of osteoporosis	

The condensed skills

		☑ or score (1–5)
Communication skills	Talking sensitively with women about sexuality and other intimate issues	
Examination skills	Breast examination	
	Pelvic examination (including digital and speculum examination, assessment of the size, position and mobility of the uterus, and the recognition of abnormality of the pelvic organs)	
	Use of obstetric Doppler (e.g. Sonicaid) or foetal stethoscope	
	Tip: *Always pay attention to professional etiquette, providing information, obtaining informed consent and patient comfort*	
Procedures	Female catheterisation	
	Change a ring pessary	
	Taking and fixing a cervical sample for liquid-based cytology (LBC)	
Self-awareness and reflective skills	Identifying own values, attitudes and approach to ethical issues affecting women (e.g. abortion, contraception for minors, consent, confidentiality, cosmetic surgery)	

The condensed know-how

	☑ or score (1–5)
Primary care management of women's risk factors, health problems, conditions and diseases. **Tip:** *Consider studying for the Diploma of the Royal College of Obstetricians and Gynaecologists (RCOG), especially if you have a secondary care O&G post*	
The indications for urgent referral to specialist services, for patients with breast lumps, gynaecological or obstetric emergencies. **Tip:** *Find out how to obtain urgent early pregnancy scans and assessment*	
Screening and case-finding strategies relevant to women (e.g. cervical, breast, other cancers, postnatal depression) and their advantages/ disadvantages, and tensions between the science and politics of screening. **Tip:** *Review the Edinburgh Postnatal Depression Scale[36] for assessing mood in postnatal women*	
Prevention strategies relevant to women (e.g. safer sex, pre-pregnancy counselling, antenatal care, immunisation, osteoporosis) and issues around health promotion, and the impact of this on the unborn child, growing children and the family	
Awareness of local support services, referral services, networks and groups for women. **Tip:** *Familiarise yourself with local family planning services, breast cancer nurses and domestic violence resources*	
The issues around equity and access to information and health services for women, practice management issues affecting the provision of care to women including availability of female doctors and informing patients of results of screening and ensuring follow-up, and the role of well-woman clinics. **Tip:** *Evaluate the effectiveness of the primary care service you provide from the female patient's point of view*	
Ability to question sensitively and safely about domestic violence and respond appropriately. **Tip:** *See the condensed resources below*	

Continued over

	☑ or score (1–5)
Confidentiality issues that relate to women (family issues, domestic violence, termination of pregnancy, sexually transmitted infections and 'Partner Notification'). **Tip:** *The GMC guidance* Confidentiality *(2009) is available on the GMC website at: www.gmc-uk.org/guidance/ethical_guidance/confidentiality.asp*	
The issues relating to the use of chaperones in women's health care. **Tip:** *Review the arrangements your practice has for providing chaperones*	
The issues of gender and power, and the effect of this on the doctor–patient relationship	
The impact of culture and ethnicity on women's perceived role in society and their attendant health beliefs, and how to tailor your practice accordingly	
The psychosocial component of women's health and the need, in some cases, to provide women patients with additional emotional and organisational support (e.g. in relation to pregnancy options, HRT, breast cancer and return to work)	
The key national guidelines that influence women's healthcare provision	
Legislation relevant to women's health (e.g. abortion, contraception). **Tip:** *Familiarise yourself with the criteria relating to termination on the 'blue form' (Certificate A)*	

The condensed resources

- NICE clinical guidelines relevant to this section include *Antenatal and Postnatal Mental Health, Antenatal Care, Diabetes in Pregnancy, Familial Breast Cancer, Fertility, Heavy Menstrual Bleeding, Hypertension in Pregnancy, Ovarian Cancer, Postnatal Care, Pregnancy and Complex Social Factors* and *Urinary Incontinence*. Available at: http://guidance.nice.org.uk/CG/Published.

- NICE Public Health Guidance relevant to this section includes *Maternal and Child Nutrition*.

- SIGN guidelines relevant to this section include *Management of Perinatal Mood Disorders, Management of Suspected Bacterial Urinary Tract Infection in Adults, Management of Urinary Incontinence in Primary Care* and *Investigation of Post-menopausal Bleeding*. Available at: www.sign.ac.uk/guidelines.

- *e*-GP contains RCGP e-learning sessions on a wide range of women's health and pregnancy-related topics: www.e-GP.org.

- The RCGP online course 'Violence against women and children' provides a practical introduction to safely asking about and responding to domestic violence (www.elearning.rcgp.org.uk).

- RCOG has issued a number of relevant guidelines: www.rcog.org.uk/guidelines.

- The National Screening Committee (www.screening.nhs.uk) and NHS Cancer Screening Programmes (www.cancerscreening.nhs.uk) websites contain guidelines on screening for breast, cervical and ovarian cancer.

- Visit www.domesticviolence.co.uk for domestic violence information and support.

Statement 3.07: *Men's Health*

Overall, men experience more ill health than women and their life expectancy is around five years lower. Men tend to take more risks with their health and have higher rates of alcohol misuse, smoking, poor diet, sexually transmitted diseases and accidents. Consultation rates are lower in men than women, and these rates have declined further in recent years. Men also have a higher risk of committing suicide compared with women.

The condensed knowledge

		☑ or score (1–5)
Symptoms	Abdominal, loin and pelvic pains in men	
	Erectile dysfunction	
	Haematuria	
	Retention of urine	
	Sore/painful penis, ulceration, skin changes	
	Testicular lumps	
	Testicular pain (orchialgia)	
	Urinary symptoms: dysuria, frequency, nocturia, poor stream, prostatism	
Conditions	Male-only conditions, including:	
	• benign prostatic hypertrophy (BPH) and prostatitis	
	• circumcision (religious and non-religious)	
	• male sterilisation: vasectomy	
	• male infertility	
	• male-specific cancers: testicular and prostate cancer	
	• mental health issues including depression and suicide	

		☑ **or score (1–5)**
Conditions	• other scrotal conditions, e.g. cryptorchidism, varicocele, hydrocele, epididymal cysts, epididymo-orchitis and epididymitis	
	• sexual dysfunction including psychosexual conditions, premature ejaculation and erectile dysfunction	
	Non-sex-specific conditions that present differently in men (e.g. depression), or occur more frequently or earlier (e.g. cardiovascular disease, inguinal hernia)	
	Conditions with a lower prevalence in men that may be overlooked (e.g. osteoporosis, breast cancer)	
Investigation	Urinalysis, MSU and dipstick	
	Blood tests including renal function tests and prostate-specific antigen (PSA) test	
	Semen analysis	
	Knowledge of secondary care investigations including prostate biopsy and testicular ultrasound	
Treatment	Understand principles of treatment for common conditions managed largely in primary care – benign prostatic hypertrophy, prostatitis, sexual dysfunction, infertility, etc.	
	Use of anti-androgens in male cancers	
Emergencies	Acute management of testicular torsion	
	Acute management of paraphimosis and priapism	
	Acute urinary retention	
	Acute management of ureteric colic	
Prevention	Health education regarding lifestyle and risk-taking behaviour, sexual and mental health	

The condensed skills

		☑ **or score** **(1–5)**
Communication skills	Developing a non-judgemental, caring and professional consulting style to maximise accessibility and minimise embarrassment	
	Techniques for compensating, when necessary, for men being less articulate about their health	
	Encouraging men to express and modify their health beliefs	
Examination skills	Testicular examination	
	Digital rectal examination	
	Tip: *Always pay attention to professional etiquette, providing information, obtaining informed consent and patient comfort*	
Procedures	Male catheterisation	
	Insertion of anti-androgen implants	
Risk management	Understanding that violence and aggression are more common among young men, how to assess the risk of harm to the patient, yourself and others, and manage this safely	

The condensed know-how

	☑ **or score** **(1–5)**
Primary care management of men's risk factors, health problems, conditions and diseases (and the relative prevalence of medical conditions in men compared with women), including men with genito-urinary problems	
The impact of male gender on health beliefs and lifestyle, and the changing gender roles to which men are expected to conform, and strategies for responding to these	
The impact of illness, in both the male patient and his family, on the presentation and management of men's health problems. **Tip:** *Remember that self-employed people and those on short-term contracts may only receive statutory sick pay*	
Screening strategies relevant to men, the indications for a PSA blood test, its role in the diagnosis and management of prostate cancer, the arguments for and against a national PSA screening programme. **Tip:** *www.cancerscreening.nhs.uk/prostate/informationpack.html has useful information, including patient information leaflets, on PSA screening*	
Health promotion and disease prevention strategies (e.g. safe sex) for men and techniques for opportunistic health education during consultations with infrequent attenders. **Tip:** *Consider the role of the practice nurse in delivering effective health promotion for men*	
The indications for urgent referral to specialist services, for patients with emergencies including testicular lumps and suspected testicular cancer. **Tip:** *Review the NICE guidelines on referral for suspected cancer (www.nice.org.uk)*	
How men's typical consulting patterns vary from women's and, as a result, how online booking systems, appointments outside the working week, email and telephone consultations may particularly improve accessibility for male patients	
Understanding that male patients may have preferences for seeing a male or female GP for certain conditions and strategies for accommodating these	
The particular difficulties that adolescent and young adult males have when accessing primary care services and ways to address this	

Continued over

	☑ **or score (1–5)**
How relationships with male patients will differ depending on the gender of the doctor, and how and when to re-establish boundaries in the doctor–patient relationship	
How cultural background may affect a man's attitudes towards health, expectations of the doctor, and presentation	
Understanding of the specific health needs of male groups, including:	
• fathers	
• gay, bisexual and transgender men	
• black and minority ethnic men	
• unemployed men	
The features of a successful men's health service, including social and cultural factors. **Tip:** Evaluate the effectiveness of the primary care service you provide from the male patient's point of view	
Practical ways of engaging men more effectively with their health (e.g. male-targeted programmes and resources)	
National guidance and legislation of relevance to men's health	

The condensed resources

> **Understanding men's health involves three main themes:** [37]
>
> - biological determinants
> - lifestyle and individual risk taking
> - masculinity and socialisation.

- NICE clinical guidelines relevant to this section include *Lower Urinary Tract Symptoms* and *Prostate Cancer*. Available at: http://guidance.nice.org.uk/CG/Published.

- SIGN guidelines relevant to this section include *Management of Suspected Bacterial Urinary Tract Infection in Adults* and *Management of Urinary Incontinence in Primary Care*. Available at: www.sign.ac.uk/guidelines.

- The evidence-based journal *Bandolier* has an interesting men's health collection: www.medicine.ox.ac.uk/bandolier/booth/booths/men.html.

- The Men's Health Forum (www.menshealthforum.org.uk) promotes men's health policy development (including Men's Health Week) and runs a site providing health advice aimed at men: www.malehealth.co.uk.

- The International Society of Men's Health provides relevant publications and a forum for exchanging information on men's health issues: www.ismh.org.

- The website www.embarrassingproblems.com is a useful resource to direct embarrassed male teenagers (and adults!).

Statement 3.08: *Sexual Health*

GPs have an important role in the management of sexual health problems, including sexually transmitted infections (STIs), human immunodeficiency virus (HIV) diagnosis, contraception, unwanted pregnancy and sexual dysfunction. Primary healthcare teams are ideally placed to take a holistic and integrated approach to sexual health, which is a UK health priority. GP education should promote integrated learning about sexual health within the complex teams and systems of the NHS.

The condensed knowledge

		☑ or score (1–5)
Symptoms	Abnormal genital smell	
	Genital skin conditions including rashes, lumps, ulcers and lichen sclerosis	
	Intermenstrual bleeding	
	Lower abdominal pain in women	
	Pain on intercourse	
	Pain on passing urine in men and women	
	Testicular and scrotal pain and swellings	
	Penile urethral discharge or different vaginal discharge	
	Vaginal bleeding after sex	
Conditions	Ano-genital ulcers – herpes simplex, syphilis, primary HIV infection	
	Ano-genital warts	
	Bacterial vaginosis	
	Candidiasis	

		☑ **or score** **(1–5)**
Conditions	Chlamydial infections	
	Conditions suggestive of immunosuppression (e.g. pneumocystis, pneumonia, tuberculosis, lymphoma, seborrhoeic dermatitis or oral thrush) or of primary HIV infection	
	Conjunctivitis (neonatal and adult).	
	Gonorrhoea	
	Group B haemolytic streptococcus. **Tip:** *Familiarise yourself with your local protocol on antenatal screening for Group B strep*	
	HIV and acquired immune deficiency syndrome (AIDS) and the presentations/complications including pneumocystis pneumonia, candidiasis, cryptococcus, Kaposi's sarcoma, toxoplasmosis, lymphoma, hepatitis, tuberculosis	
	Reiter's syndrome (reactive arthritis)	
	Sexual dysfunction	
	Sexual identity disorders and gender realignment	
	Syphilis	
	Trichomonas vaginalis	
Investigation	Pregnancy testing	
	Urinalysis, MSU and dipstick	
	Blood tests for HIV and appropriate counselling	
	Blood tests for syphilis and their interpretation	
	Blood tests for hepatitis B and their interpretation	
	Microbiology and virology swabs from genitalia and throat – which to use, which samples to take, limitations of tests and interpretation of results	
	Awareness of secondary care investigations, e.g. colposcopy	

Continued over

		☑ **or score** **(1–5)**
Emergencies	Ectopic pregnancy and miscarriage	
	Emergency contraception	
	Infection in the immune-compromised patient	
	Post-HIV exposure prophylaxis	
	Severe pelvic inflammatory disease	
	Sexual assault or rape	
Treatment	Contraception – effectiveness rates, risks, benefits and appropriate selection of patients for all methods, including oral and intrauterine methods of emergency contraception. **Tip:** *Information on all methods can be found on the Family Planning Association (FPA) website: www.fpa.org.uk*	
	Hormonal contraception – the safe provision of all methods of oral contraception (including emergency hormonal contraception) and contraceptive patches/rings. **Tip:** *The* UK Medical Eligibility Criteria for Contraceptive Use *guidelines are available at: www.fsrh.org/pages/clinical_guidance.asp*	
	Long-acting reversible contraception (LARC) – benefits, risks and availability of LARC methods of contraception including intrauterine methods, DMPA injections and subdermal implants	
	Other methods of contraception – including barrier methods, natural methods, vasectomy and sterilisation	
	Abortion – methods and the legal procedures relating to referral for abortion. **Tip:** *Find out the local counselling and clinical arrangements for women requesting termination of pregnancy*	

		☑ or score (1–5)
Treatment	Principles of treatment for common conditions diagnosed and/or managed in primary care (see above) and common patterns of antibiotic resistance (e.g. gonorrhoea)	
	Principles of antiretroviral combination therapy for HIV/AIDS, potential side effects and the role of the GP in shared-care management	
Prevention	Emergency contraception after unprotected sex	
	Health education and prevention programmes (e.g. safer sex and risk reduction)	
	Hepatltis B vaccination	
	HPV vaccination	
	National screening programmes (e.g. antenatal HIV testing, cervlcal screening, chlamydia)	

The condensed skills

		☑ or score (1–5)
Consultation skills	Techniques for sensitively raising sexual health issues opportunistically in a consultation	
Counselling skills	Counselling patients with sexual problems including psychosexual issues related to contraception, sexually transmitted infection, HIV testing, and for patients who have an unplanned or unwanted pregnancy	
Examination skills	Performing a sexual health examination including digital and speculum examination.	
	Tip: *Always pay attention to professional etiquette, giving information, consent and patient comfort*	
Procedures	Giving an intramuscular injection	
	Taking microbiology and virology swabs (from ano-genital areas and throat), storage and transport	
	Teaching a patient about male and female condom use	

Continued over

		☑ or score (1–5)
Risk assessment skills	Assessing risk and tailoring advice and care accordingly	
Self-awareness and reflective skills	Ensuring that your own beliefs, moral or religious reservations about any contraceptive methods, abortion or sexual behaviours do not adversely affect your patient's care	
Sexual history-taking skills **Tip:** *Attending a STIF course is a good way to practice these skills: www.bashh.org*	Taking a sexual history from a male or female patient (in a way that is confidential, non-judgemental, responsive to the patient and avoids assumptions about sexual orientation or the gender of the partner, or assumptions related to age, disability or ethnic origin)	
	Using sexual history (including partner history and information on sexual practices including condom use) and other relevant information to assess risk of STI, unwanted pregnancy and cervical cancer	
	Applying the information gathered to generate a differential diagnosis and formulate a management plan	

The condensed know-how

	☑ or score (1–5)
Understand the concept of sexual health and the GP's role in promoting this in the consultation, within his or her teams, and more widely	
The epidemiology of sexual health problems and how this is reflected in the local population. **Tip:** *Consider the sexual health needs of specific populations (e.g. students)*	
Factors affecting accessibility of sexual health services and strategies to improve this. **Tip:** *Review how accessible your practice is to young people seeking sexual health or contraception advice*	

	☑ **or score** **(1–5)**
Team-working with practice nurses, healthcare assistants, health visitors and receptionists, to ensure accessibility and coordination of sexual health services. **Tip:** *Spend time with health visitors when they are seeing patients with sexual health concerns or problems (e.g. young mothers)*	
Referral criteria and processes to local specialist services, including gynaecologists, sexual and reproductive health specialists, genito-urinary specialists, urologists, specialists in infectious diseases and specialists in sexual dysfunction. **Tip:** *Arrange an attachment to your local sexual health or genito-urinary medicine (GUM) clinic*	
Strategies for the promotion of sexual health and the early detection of sexual health problems that may have not yet produced symptoms. **Tip:** Does your practice offer chlamydia screening?	
The particular confidentiality issues related to sexual health and the policies for ensuring these are managed in your practice. **Tip:** *Find out about the doctor's duty of confidentiality and the issues raised by the Sexual Offences Act 2003 (different guidance applies in different countries in the UK)*	
A working knowledge of the functional anatomy and physiology of the male and female genital systems	
Common presentations of sexual dysfunction, and of sexual violence and abuse, including covert presentations such as somatisation	
The limitations of 'watching and waiting' in sexual health, because some serious infections (e.g. chlamydia and HIV) may lapse back into being asymptomatic and cause harm to the patient	
Techniques to explain the benefits and address inappropriate beliefs about long-acting reversible contraceptive methods, which could benefit many women. **Tip:** *Review the* UK Medical Eligibility Criteria for Contraceptive Use *at:* www.fsrh.org	
Specific interventions for HIV prevention such as post-exposure prophylaxis and the prevention of mother-to-baby transmission	

Continued over

	☑ **or score** **(1–5)**
Sexual health screening programmes in use in the UK and the benefits, limitations and need for informed consent. **Tip:** *See statement 3.01:* Healthy People: promoting health and preventing disease *for more information on the issues around screening*	
Patient groups at greater risk of unplanned pregnancies and value of opportunistic approach for health promotion and contraception advice	
Principles of and current guidance for partner notification and the issues this raises around confidentiality. **Tip:** *The GMC guidance* Confidentiality *(2009) is available on the GMC website at: www.gmc-uk.org/guidance/ethical_guidance/confidentiality.asp*	
Advice on how your patients can access local sexual health services directly, including services that provide specialist contraceptive care; termination of pregnancy; STI diagnosis and management; HIV management and services for relationship problems and sexual dysfunction **Tip:** *Consider spending a session attached to your local sexual health clinic*	
Cultural factors that affect the patient's risk of having sexual health problems and also his or her reactions to them, and the social stigma often associated with sexual health problems or sexual orientation and behaviour	
Need to address factors associated with risky sexual behaviour including mental health problems, drug and alcohol misuse, and a history of sexual abuse	
Awareness of patient groups where sexual health needs may be inappropriately omitted by health professionals (e.g. those with physical or intellectual disability, or older adults)	
Legal aspects relating to sexual health including termination of pregnancy and the methods used in the UK, and the provision of contraception and sexual health treatment to under-16s (including child safeguarding). **Tip:** *Aspects include the 'Fraser guidelines' relating to the Gillick case,*[38] *the Human Rights Act 1998 and the Sexual Offences Act 2003*	
Ethical principles involved when treating patients who have sexual health concerns (e.g. contraception and abortion)	

	☑ **or score**
	(1–5)

Key national guidelines and strategies that influence sexual healthcare provision.

Tip: *The UK government's* Teenage Pregnancy Strategy: beyond 2010 *is available on the DH website at: www.education.gov.uk/publications/ standard/publicationDetail/Page1/DCSF-00224-2010*

The condensed resources

- NICE clinical guidelines relevant to this section include *Long-Acting Reversible Contraception*. Available at: http://guidance.nice.org.uk/CG/Published.

- NICE Public Health Guidance relevant to this section includes two guidelines on increasing the uptake of HIV testing.

- SIGN guidelines relevant to this section include *Management of Genital Chlamydia Trachomatis Infection*. Available at: www.sign.ac.uk/guidelines.

- e-GP contains RCGP e-learning sessions on sexual health that cover most of the topics in this statement: www.e-GP.org.

- The RCGP Introductory Certificate in Sexual Health online course (www.elearning.rcgp.org.uk) provides an introduction to sexual health issues for GPs.

- The course for the Diploma of the Faculty of Family Planning and Reproductive Healthcare (www.ffprhc.org.uk) provides a solid foundation on sexual health and contraception. On gaining the diploma, those who wish can then progress to obtaining letters of competence in the fitting of subdermal implants (LoC SDI) and intrauterine techniques (LoC IUT).

- The charity FPA provides information on contraception and sexually transmitted infections: www.fpa.org.uk.

- The British Association for Sexual Health and HIV: www.bashh.org.

- The British Society for Sexual Medicine: www.bssm.org.uk.

- The Terrence Higgins Trust provides a wide range of publications and information on HIV, AIDS and sexual health for health professionals and the public: www.tht.org.uk.

- College of Sexual and Relationship Therapists (COSRT): www.cosrt.org.uk.

- Relate offers a psychosexual counselling service in addition to its relationship counselling services: www.relate.org.uk.

- The International Planned Parenthood Foundation (www.ippf.org) has a free directory listing the drugs contained in non-UK-sourced contraceptive pills.

Statement 3.09: *End-of-Life Care*

GPs are responsible for the end-of-life care of both cancer and non-cancer patients. Enabling patients to die with dignity and with minimal distress is one of the most fundamental aspects of medicine. Many terminally ill patients prefer the option of a peaceful death at home and the primary care team has a crucial role to play in enabling this to happen, in supporting the patient and his or her carers through the process, and in providing care for the family after the death has occurred.

The condensed knowledge

		☑ or score (1–5)
Emergencies	Acute anxiety/panic or agitation	
	Dysphagia	
	Hypercalcaemia	
	Major haemorrhage	
	Pathological bone fractures	
	Spinal cord compression	
	Superior vena caval obstruction	
Treatment	Management of distressing symptoms:	
	• agitation and anxiety	
	• breathlessness	
	• confusion	
	• constipation	
	• nausea and vomiting	
	• pain	
	Tip: *Learn the World Health Organization (WHO) pain relief ladder: www.who.int/cancer/palliative/painladder*	

Continued over

		☑ **or score (1–5)**
Treatment	Knowledge about a syringe driver:	
	● indications	
	● writing up suitable drugs, doses and combinations	
	● conversion of drugs from oral dosage to syringe drive, either IV or subcutaneous	
	● managing complications (e.g. breakthrough pain, local reactions)	
	Tip: *Read the BNF section on 'Prescribing in Palliative Care'*	
	Use of emergency drugs in palliative care	

The condensed skills

		☑ **or score (1–5)**
Communication skills	Communicating sensitively and effectively with the patient and carer(s) regarding difficult information about the disease, its progression or its prognosis	
Counselling skills	Advising, motivating and explaining:	
	● stage and progression of disease	
	● prognosis	
	● symptom control and management options	
	● what to expect	
	● advance care planning	
	● processes relating to death and dying	
	● bereavement	
Leadership and team-working skills	Functioning both as leader and proactive member of end-of-life care teams as required	

	☑ or score (1–5)
Procedures — Setting up a syringe driver	
Reflective and housekeeping skills — Addressing your personal attitudes and experiences that can affect your attitude towards patients with terminal conditions or who are dying	

The condensed know-how

	☑ or score (1–5)
The principles of palliative care and how they apply to both cancer and non-cancer illnesses such as cardiovascular, neurological, respiratory and infectious diseases. **Tip:** *Remember that people with non-cancer terminal conditions (e.g. heart failure, severe COPD) deserve high-quality end-of-life care too*	
The NHS Gold Standards Framework for end-of-life care and how to apply this to your own practice as both a clinician and a team leader	
Practical ways of providing person-centred care that considers the physical, psychological, social and spiritual needs of the patient, his or her carers and family	
Factors affecting the provision of 24-hour continuity of care through various clinical systems. **Tip:** *Find out how to notify your local out-of-hours service about palliative and terminally ill patients*	
The social benefits and services available to patients and carers. **Tip:** *Find out the rules on the DS1500 form for accessing benefits quickly for the terminally ill*	
The health, economic, social and psychological impacts of caring for a dying patient on that patient's family, friends, dependants and employers. **Tip:** *Find out how to arrange respite care or overnight nursing*	
The normal and abnormal grieving process and its impact upon symptomatology. **Tip:** *Well-recognised bereavement models include the phases of grief, tasks of mourning, dimensions of loss and dual-process models*	

Continued over

	☑ or score (1–5)
The key health service policy documents and guidelines that influence provision for cancer and palliative care. **Tip:** *The NICE 'End of life care' quality standard is available at: www.nice.org.uk/guidance/qualitystandards/endoflifecare/home.jsp*	
Ethical and legal dimensions of treatment and investigation choices, palliative and terminal care, euthanasia and advanced directives	

The condensed resources

- The NHS Gold Standards Framework for end-of-life care can be accessed at: www.goldstandardsframework.org.uk.

- Palliative Care Guidelines for Scotland: www.palliativecareguidelines.scot.nhs.uk.

- The GMC's *Treatment and Care Towards the End of Life: good practice in decision making* (2010) is available at: www.gmc-uk.org/guidance/ethical_guidance/end_of_life_care.asp.

- Liverpool Care Pathway: www.liv.ac.uk/mcpcil/liverpool-care-pathway.

- *e*-GP contains RCGP e-learning sessions on pain and symptom control, the final days, and ethical, psychosocial and medico-legal issues at the end of life: www.e-GP.org.

- e-Learning for healthcare end-of-life programme: www.e-elca.org.uk.

- Cruse Bereavement Care offers advice on the normal bereavement process and provides counselling and support to people who have been bereaved: www.crusebereavementcare.org.uk.

- Marie Curie Cancer Care provides free nursing care to terminally ill people to give them the choice of dying at home: www.mariecurie.org.uk.

- Palliative Care Matters website: www.pallcare.info.

Resources about cancer (but not necessarily end-of-life) care include the following:

- cancer statistics are available from the Cancer Research UK website: www.cancerresearchuk.org/cancerstats

- Macmillan Cancer Support offers support to patients with cancer and produces advice leaflets: www.macmillan.org.uk

- NICE clinical guidance on *Referral for Suspected Cancer* is available at: http://guidance.nice.org.uk/CG27

- a summary of the NHS Cancer Strategy for England is available at: www.ncat.nhs.uk.

Statement 3.10: *Care of People with Mental Health Problems*

Promoting mental health resilience and providing care for people with mental health problems is integral to the work of a GP and has implications for the public health of the practice population. Mental health problems seen in primary care include a large range of conditions. In particular, GPs should be able to recognise depression and anxiety, and assess its severity; patients with mental health problems should be screened for suicide and self-harm risks, and safeguarding concerns should be considered for children and vulnerable adults. People with severe mental illness have a high prevalence of physical co-morbidity that must also be managed.

GPs should be aware that all physical illness has a psychological component; this should be taken into account in management plans. Developing skills to recognise and manage somatisation could save patient suffering and healthcare costs. Communication skills and patient-centred practice are highly important in improving the recognition and effective management of mental health problems.

The condensed knowledge

		☑ or score (1–5)
Symptoms	Anxiety	
	Depression	
	Early features of psychotic illness	
	Hyperventilation (e.g. breathlessness, dizziness, palpitations and paraesthesiae)	
	Sleep disorders	
	Somatic complaints (e.g. abdominal pain, headache)	
	Tired all the time (if physical causes excluded)	

		☑ **or score (1–5)**
Conditions	Attention deficit hyperactivity disorder (ADHD)	
	Alcohol and drug misuse (see condensed statement 3.14)	
	Anxiety disorders (including generalised anxiety, panic attacks, social anxiety, phobias)	
	Bereavement reaction	
	Depression	
	Eating disorders	
	Obsessive-compulsive disorder	
	Personality disorders	
	Post-traumatic stress disorder	
	Schizophrenia and psychotic illness	
	Somatisation disorder	
Investigation	Use of Whooley questions [39] for case-finding in patients with long-term conditions.	
	Tip: *The two questions are: 'During the past month, have you often been bothered by feeling down, depressed or hopeless?' and 'During the past month, have you often been bothered by having little interest or pleasure in doing things?' A positive response to either question requires further assessment*	
	Use of validated rating scales (e.g. PHQ-9 and GAD-7), and other aids to evaluation of possible diagnosis and severity (see condensed resources below)	
Treatment	Drug treatments	
	Cognitive behavioural therapy (CBT) and simple behavioural techniques	
	Problem-solving therapy	
	Psychodynamic psychotherapies	
	Self-administered therapy	

Continued over

		☑ or score (1–5)
Emergency	Threatened or attempted suicide	
	Delirium	
	Psychosis	
	Panic	
	Aggressive or violent patients	
	Drug overdose and alcohol withdrawal	
Prevention	Concepts of mental health promotion, especially for children, young people and families	
	Early intervention in psychosis	
	Screening of all language-delayed children for autism	
	Supporting patients to remain in and return to work and avoid long-term worklessness	

The condensed skills

		☑ or score (1–5)
Consultation skills	Establishing rapport with the patient, his or her carers and family, and maintaining a good relationship in challenging circumstances	
	Enabling patients to disclose their concerns and using case-finding and assessment tools in a patient-centred way	
	Negotiating an appropriate and acceptable shared management plan and integrating physical, psychological and social ideas and plans	
	Avoiding medicalising common mental distresses and dealing appropriately with the uncertainty that certain patients may produce	
	Responding quickly and appropriately to concerns raised by carers, relatives and others	

		☑ or score (1–5)
Cognitive skills	Mental state assessment	
	Suicide risk assessment	
Self-awareness and reflective skills	Self-awareness and reflective skills. These are needed to develop a personal management plan for your own mental health and to understand how your own attitudes and feelings affect how you manage patients who:	
	• self-harm	
	• use services chaotically	
	• know more about their illnesses than their doctors do	
	• engender strong emotions	

The condensed know-how

	☑ or score (1–5)
The prevalence of mental health problems and needs among the practice population and any relevant local health improvement programmes	
The principles of mental health promotion and the concept of 'resilience'	
The diagnostic criteria for the common mental health problems seen in primary care	
How to screen for mental illness, using effective and reliable instruments, and issues around the screening and diagnosis of people with physical illness	
Evidence-based management of mental health problems in primary care, including different forms of talking therapy, medication and self-help, based on a stepped-care model. **Tip:** *Find out how your patients can access the Improving Access to Psychological Therapies programme, which provides talking treatments (e.g. self-help, problem solving, CBT, psychodynamic psychotherapy, supportive counselling)*	
Specific evidence-based interventions and best practice for individual mental health conditions, as described in the SIGN or NICE guidelines	

Continued over

	☑ **or score** **(1–5)**
Early indicators of psychological difficulties in children and young people, including ways that a first episode of psychosis may present in the young, and how to respond to this promptly and effectively	
Issues around frequent attenders, patients who demand drugs, and chronic suicidal traits in borderline personality disorder. **Tip:** *Discuss various strategies for managing 'demanding' patients in your learning group*	
Psychosomatic complaints, psychological consequences of physical illness and somatisation, and the challenges of avoiding under- and over-investigation	
How to access mental health and social care organisations that support people with mental health problems, both voluntary and statutory. **Tip:** *Find out about the local mental health service arrangements in your area, especially the phone numbers of the local mental health crisis teams and who to refer to 'out of hours'*	
Indications for referral to specialist mental health services	
Responsibilities for safeguarding and supporting children and young people in difficulty, and how to access support and advice from specialist child and adolescent mental health services (CAMHS)	
The concept of concordance; how it is particularly important in mental health care and how presenting individuals with choices can improve the effectiveness of intervention	
The particular issues around continuity of care for people with mental health problems and the importance of an integrated approach. **Tip:** *Find out about the Care Programme Approach (CPA) and the role of the key worker or care coordinator*	
The commonly associated physical health problems of people with mental health problems. **Tip:** *Particular problems involve lifestyle issues including smoking, drug misuse, weight disorders and difficulties using health services appropriately*	
The impact of social circumstances on mental illness and recovery, the negative impact of social exclusion, and the principles of promoting recovery	

	☑ **or score** **(1–5)**
The extent and implications of stigma and social exclusion relating to mental illness. **Tip:** *You can learn about patients' experiences of living with mental illness at: www.healthtalkonline.org*	
Cultural determinants of mental illness, the use of value judgements in psychiatric diagnosis and the problems caused by assumptions that may not be universally held (e.g. that a condition is physical not psychological)	
Being prepared to work with other agencies in promoting mental health in your local community	
Ethical issues around compulsory treatment and the inappropriate use of psychotropic drugs to sedate people for nursing or social reasons	
Sufficient knowledge of the current Mental Health Act and the responsibilities of a GP in relation to this. **Tip:** *Learn about the role of the approved social worker and try to attend a Mental Health Act assessment at least once during your training*	

The condensed resources

- NICE clinical guidelines relevant to this section include *Antenatal and Postnatal Mental Health, Antisocial Personality Disorder, Anxiety, ADHD, Autism in Children and Young People, Bipolar Disorder, Borderline Personality Disorder, Chronic Fatigue Syndrome* and *Common Mental Health Disorders*, plus several guidelines on *Depression, Eating Disorders, Obsessive Compulsive Disorder and Body Dysmorphic Disorder, Post-traumatic Stress Disorder, Psychosis with Coexisting Substance Misuse, Schizophrenia* and *Self-harm*. Available at: http://guidance.nice.org.uk/CG/Published.

- NICE quality standard for depression in adults is available at: www.nice.org.uk/guidance/qualitystandards/depressioninadults/home.jsp.

- SIGN guidelines relevant to this section include *Management of Perinatal Mood Disorders, Non-pharmaceutical Management of Depression* and *Bipolar Affective Disorder*. Available at: www.sign.ac.uk/guidelines.

- The RCGP 'Improving access to psychological therapies' online course introduces the stepped-care approach and explains the evidence-based treatment of common mental health problems: www.elearning.rcgp.org.uk.

- The RCGP online course 'Mental health in older people' considers the challenges of managing mental health problems in older patients: www.elearning.rcgp.org.uk.

- The Healthy Working UK website contains information, resources and advice for healthcare practitioners on 'fit notes' and supporting patients returning to work: www.healthyworkinguk.co.uk.

- The Royal College of Psychiatrists provides information and guidance on mental health issues: www.rcpsych.ac.uk.

- The PHQ-9 (Patient Health Questionnaire) and GAD-7 (Generalised Anxiety Disorder) assessments can be accessed via: www.patient.co.uk.

- A summary of the Mental Health Act 1983 can be found on the Department for Work and Pensions website at: www.dwp.gov.uk/publications/specialist-guides/medical-conditions/mental-health-act.shtml.

- An overview of the NSF for Mental health can be found at: www.nhs.uk/NHSEngland/NSF/Pages/Mentalhealth.aspx.

Statement 3.11: *Care of People with Intellectual Disability*

There are over 200,000 people in the UK living with an intellectual disability. People with intellectual disability have an increased level of morbidity and mortality, and GPs must be aware of the most likely associated conditions and where to obtain specialist help and advice. GPs must also understand how psychiatric and physical illness may present atypically in patients with sensory, communication and cognitive difficulties. Additional skills of communication, diagnosis and examination are needed to care for patients who have difficulties with describing or verbalising their symptoms.

The condensed knowledge

		☑ or score (1–5)
Symptoms	Diagnostic overshadowing is common; this is where a symptom is incorrectly attributed to the intellectual disability rather than the true cause. Common symptoms that might be due to another underlying health condition include:	
	• agitation	
	• challenging behaviour	
	• tearfulness	
	• weight loss and gain	
	• withdrawal	
Conditions	Cerebral palsy	
	Dermatological problems	
	Epilepsy – increased incidence and complexity associated with increased severity of learning disability	
	Gastrointestinal (GI) – swallowing problems, reflux oesophagitis, *Helicobacter pylori*, constipation	
	Obesity – predisposes to other health problems, stigma	
	Orthopaedic problems – joint contractures, osteoporosis	

Continued over

		☑ **or score (1–5)**
Conditions	Psychiatric problems – emotional and behavioural disorders, schizophrenia, bipolar affective disorder, Alzheimer's disease in Down's syndrome	
	Respiratory problems – chest infections, aspiration pneumonia	
	Sensory impairments – hearing and vision disorders, earwax	
	Sexual and physical abuse	
Treatment	Hurdles in the delivery of treatment due to difficulties reading instructions and treatment labels	
	The risks of 'over the counter' medications for some patients who may not fully understand how or why to take treatments but live with some degree of independence	
	Issues around implementation of interventions – e.g. dependency on carers, the difficulties with drug delivery in residential care homes	
	Difficulties around identifying drug side effects	
Emergency	In urgent life-threatening cases treatment needs to proceed in the best interests of a person with insufficient capacity to consent	
Resources	Specialist learning disability teams and non-medical agencies	
Prevention	Health reviews proposed for people with intellectual disability	

The condensed skills

		☑ or score (1–5)
Coordination of care skills	Addressing barriers to health care for people with intellectual disability including a lack of appropriate support services (e.g. behavioural support, psychiatric or neurological assessment services), especially during the transition from adolescence to adulthood	
Consultation skills	Communicating effectively with patients with sensory difficulties and providing information in an appropriate format	
	Maintaining a patient-centred approach while communicating with carers and respecting the patient's autonomy, being aware how communication with carers may skew the doctor–patient relationship (e.g. difficulty raising personal issues, such as sexual or mental health)	
Time-management skills	Providing more time in the consultation to manage people with intellectual disability more effectively	

The condensed know-how

	☑ or score (1–5)
The scientific evidence regarding the health needs of people with intellectual disability, in the following areas:	
• untreated, yet treatable, medical conditions	
• untreated specific health issues related to the individual's disability	
• a lack of uptake of generic (non-targeted) health promotion	
The difficulties faced by patients with mild intellectual disability, who may need no particular special services, but who may have reading, writing and comprehension difficulties.	
Tip: *Arrange an attachment with a community speech and language therapist*	

Continued over

	☑ **or score (1–5)**
The difficulties faced by patients with moderate, severe and profound intellectual disability who have special needs for accessing services and need to be identified, monitored and reviewed appropriately. **Tip:** *Do a case study on a patient in your practice with intellectual disability and the challenges he or she faces*	
The likely conditions associated with intellectual disability, their common medical problems and where to obtain specialist help and advice. **Tip:** *Find out about your local enablement centre and the services it provides*	
Techniques to optimise communication through the use of communication aids, and the impact of the doctor's working environment on patient care (e.g. the measures that should be taken to compensate for sensory impairment)	
The particular issues around equitable access to services and information, and maintaining continuity of care in patients with intellectual disability	
How psychiatric and physical illness may present atypically in patients with intellectual disability who have sensory, communication and cognitive difficulties. **Tip:** *Consider the impact of 'diagnostic overshadowing', when a doctor incorrectly assumes a person's symptoms are due to his or her learning disability rather than an alternative underlying cause*	
How to use additional enquiry, appropriate tests and careful examination in patients unable to describe or verbalise symptoms	
The importance of health promotion in people with learning difficulties and the challenges in doing this effectively	
The requirements of the NHS annual health check for people with intellectual disability	
The roles of carers, respite care opportunities, day centres and voluntary and statutory agencies, and how you can support unpaid carers in your own practice. **Tip:** *Find out about Attendance Allowance and Disability Living Allowance and your potential role in supporting patients to apply for these*	

	☑ **or score**
	(1–5)

The impact of intellectual disability on family dynamics and the implications for physical, psychological and social morbidity in the patient's carers and the GP's role in providing carer health promotion and support	
The particular issues around capacity and consent, and the mechanisms by which these can be determined and enhanced. **Tip:** *Information on this and on the Mental Capacity Act 2005 is available at: www.justice.gov.uk/about/opg*	
The effects of prejudice and unfair discrimination on people with learning difficulties and the duty of GPs to recognise this within themselves, others and practice systems, and take remedial action	

The condensed resources

- The RCGP has produced a toolkit to support GPs carrying out annual health checks for people with intellectual disability (www.rcgp.org.uk).

- *e*-GP contains a programme of RCGP e-learning sessions on caring for people with intellectual disability (www.e-GP.org).

- Directgov provides information for disabled people on employment, financial support, accessibility and rights: www.direct.gov.uk/en/DisabledPeople/index.htm.

- The British Institute of Learning Disabilities (BILD) supports people with intellectual disability and their families: www.bild.org.uk.

- The National Autistic Society offers information for health professionals on diagnosing autism and Asperger's syndrome: www.autism.org.uk.

- The GMC website has an area devoted to learning disabilities: www.gmc-uk.org/learningdisabilities.

- Reports on learning disability, including *Nothing About Us Without Us* and *Valuing People*, are available at: www.publications.doh.gov.uk/learningdisabilities/access.

Statement 3.12: *Cardiovascular Health*

Cardiovascular problems are a major cause of morbidity and mortality in the UK; around 50% of 45-year-olds subsequently die from coronary heart disease so management of the risk factors in the mid- to latter stages of life is an essential part of health promotion in general practice. Primary and secondary prevention of cardiovascular disease, and associated chronic kidney disease, occurs mainly in primary care and has significant clinical benefit. GPs should be competent at managing cardiovascular emergencies and accurately diagnosing symptoms that may be due to cardiovascular causes.

The condensed knowledge

		☑ or score (1–5)
Symptoms	Ankle swelling	
	Breathlessness	
	Chest pain	
	Collapses, dizziness or faints	
	Palpitations and silent arrhythmias	
	Relating to cerebrovascular disease	
	Relating to peripheral vascular disease	
Conditions	Aneurysms (e.g. abdominal aortic aneurysm [AAA], femoral)	
	Arrhythmias (especially ectopic beats, atrial fibrillation and flutter, common tachycardias, bradyarrhythmias)	
	Cerebrovascular disease (transient ischaemic attack [TIA] and stroke)	
	Chronic kidney disease (CKD)	
	Coronary heart disease (angina, acute myocardial infarction [MI], cardiac arrest)	
	Heart failure	
	Hypertension (essential and malignant)	

		☑ **or score** **(1–5)**
Conditions	Other less common but serious cardiac conditions (cardiomyopathy, valve problems, congenital heart disease)	
	Peripheral vascular disease (arterial and venous)	
	Thromboembolism	
Investigation	Interpretation of routine blood and urine tests for cardiovascular risk assessment and treatment monitoring (e.g. lipids and cholesterol, fasting glucose, HbA1c, eGFR, U&Es, LFTs, ACR)	
	12-lead ECG (interpreting and performing)	
	24-hour ambulatory BP	
	Indications for exercise/stress ECG, echocardiography, 24-hour ECG/event recorder and local arrangements for obtaining these	
	Venous dopplers and ankle-brachial pressure index (ABPI)	
	Awareness of common secondary care procedures (e.g. cardioversion, ablation, angiography and stenting, pacemaker fitting, CABG, valve replacement)	
Treatment	Management of patients at cardiovascular risk, especially blood pressure and lipid management	
	Chronic disease management of those with established disease	
Emergencies	Emergency care of MI, cardiac arrest, stroke and critical ischaemia	
Prevention	The role of health promotion and lifestyle interventions	
	Management of cardiovascular risk factors both modifiable (BP, lipids, smoking, alcohol, exercise, obesity, diet) and fixed (ethnicity, sex, family history)	
	Management of relevant co-morbidities (e.g. diabetes mellitus, hyperlipidaemia, CKD)	

The condensed skills

		☑ or score (1–5)
Consultation skills	Assessing and explaining the risk of cardiovascular problems clearly and effectively in a non-biased manner	
IM&T skills	Utilising disease registers and data-recording templates for opportunistic and planned monitoring of cardiovascular problems	
Examination skills	Cardiovascular examination	
Procedures	Blood pressure measurement	
	Calculation of cardiovascular risk	
	Performing an ECG and basic interpretation	

The condensed know-how

	☑ or score (1–5)
The role of other primary care health professionals (e.g. practice nurses), cardiologists and other specialists in acute and chronic cardiovascular disease management, including prevention, rehabilitation and palliative care. **Tip:** *Attend a nurse-led chronic disease management (CDM) clinic; ask about your local specialist community services*	
How to access specialist cardiovascular services, especially rapid-access chest pain clinics, specialist stroke and heart failure services	
Practice- and community-based strategies for the early detection of cardiovascular problems. **Tip:** *Review the evidence for the effectiveness of 'routine health checks' or awareness-raising initiatives in your local community (e.g. football matches). Are they effective?*	
The particular issues around non-concordance for preventive cardiovascular medicines and techniques for negotiating management	
The rationale for targeting certain investigations and treatments (e.g. open-access echocardiography, statin prescribing)	

	☑ **or score**
	(1–5)

DVLA guidelines regarding driving according to cardiovascular risks.	
Tip: *These are available on the DVLA website (www.dvla.gov.uk)*	
The social and psychological impact of cardiovascular problems on the patient, his or her family, dependants and employers, and on disability and fitness to work.	
Tip: *The British Heart Foundation produces a series of information leaflets for health professionals on this and related issues: www.bhf.org.uk*	
The cultural significance that people attach to the heart as a 'seat of emotions'	
The key government policy documents that influence healthcare provision for cardiovascular problems	
Tip: *The NICE quality standard for chronic heart failure is available at: www.nice.org.uk/guidance/qualitystandards/chronicheartfailure/home.jsp*	
The key national guidelines and research findings that influence management of cardiovascular problems (e.g. the Heart Protection Study[40])	
The ethical issues relevant to the management of cardiovascular problems (e.g. the consequences of lifestyle choices and issues of age and race).	

The condensed resources

- NICE clinical guidelines relevant to this section include *Atrial Fibrillation, Chest Pain of Recent Onset, Chronic Heart Failure, Hypertension, Lipid Modification, MI: secondary prevention, Prophylaxis against Infective Endocarditis, Stable Angina, Stroke* and *Transient Loss of Consciousness*. Available at: http://guidance.nice.org.uk/CG/Published.

- SIGN guidelines relevant to this section include *Risk Estimation and the Prevention of Cardiovascular Disease, Management of Stable Angina, Management of Chronic Heart Failure, Cardiac Arrhythmias in Coronary Heart Disease, Acute Coronary Syndromes, Cardiac Rehabilitation, Diagnosis and Management of Peripheral Arterial Disease* and *Management of Patients with Stroke or TIA*. Available at: www.sign.ac.uk/guidelines.

- The RCP's *National Clinical Guidelines for Stroke* is available at: www.rcplondon.ac.uk/resources/stroke-guidelines.

- Specific cardiovascular web resources include:

  ○ British Cardiac Society (www.bcs.com)

  ○ British Hypertension Society (www.bhsoc.org)

  ○ Primary Care Cardiovascular Society (www.pccs.org.uk)

  ○ British Heart Foundation (www.bhf.org.uk)

  ○ Stroke Association (www.stroke.org.uk).

- Cardiovascular risk prediction charts can be found in the back of the BNF; the QRISK 2-2012 calculator is available at: www.qrisk.org.

- A summary of the NSF for coronary heart disease is available at: www.nhs.uk/NHSEngland/NSF/Pages/Coronaryheartdisease.aspx.

Statement 3.13: *Digestive Health*

Digestive problems are common in general practice and most gut problems are managed in primary care. Dyspepsia and GORD are particularly common conditions, affecting around a quarter of the population. The prevention and early treatment of colorectal cancer is a UK priority, because it is the second most common cause of cancer death.

The condensed knowledge

		☑ or score (1–5)
Symptoms	Abdominal pain (including location, duration, nature, frequency, radiation and associated factors)	
	Anorexia and weight loss	
	Biliary colic	
	Change in bowel habit	
	Diarrhoea and constipation	
	Dyspeptic symptoms (e.g. bloating, epigastric pain, heartburn, regurgitation, nausea associated with meals)	
	Dysphagia	
	Haematemesis and melaena	
	Incontinence of faeces	
	Jaundice	
	Nausea and vomiting	
	Rectal bleeding	
	Tenesmus	
Conditions	Abdominal masses, organomegaly and ascites	
	Acute abdominal conditions	
	Coeliac disease and other causes of malabsorption	
	Constipation	

Continued over

		☑ **or score** **(1–5)**
Conditions	Diverticulosis	
	Gallstones and gallbladder disease	
	Gastroenteritis	
	GORD and hiatus hernia	
	GI cancers (including their red flags). **Tip:** *Refer to the NICE guidelines (www.nice.org.uk)*	
	Hepatitis (chronic viral, autoimmune and other causes)	
	Hernias (e.g. inguinal, umbilical and periumbilical, femoral, surgical), incarceration and strangulation	
	Inflammatory bowel disease (e.g. Crohn's and ulcerative colitis)	
	Irritable bowel syndrome (including making a positive diagnosis). **Tip:** *Review the Rome III criteria*[41] *for diagnosing functional bowel disorders: www.romecriteria.org*	
	Non-ulcer dyspepsia, gastritis and peptic ulceration	
	Chronic liver disease, malignancy and acute liver failure	
	Pancreatic conditions (e.g. acute and chronic pancreatitis, cancer)	
	Perianal and anal disease (e.g. fissure, haemorrhoids and tags)	
Investigation	Blood tests (liver function tests [LFTs], amylase)	
	H. pylori testing. **Tip:** *Find out what testing is available in your area and the advantages and disadvantages of the different methods*	
	Coeliac antibody screening	
	Stool testing including faecal occult bloods	
	Appropriate use of abdominal ultrasound	

		☑ or score (1–5)
Investigation	Indications and risks of common secondary care investigations (e.g. OGD endoscopy, sigmoidoscopy, barium studies, CT, liver biopsy, ERCP, jejunal biopsy)	
Treatment	Primary care management of the conditions listed in 'symptoms' and 'conditions'	
	Indications for specialist referral and awareness of secondary care management of digestive problems (medical and surgical options)	
Emergencies	Acute abdomen	
	Haematemesis and melaena	
	Incarcerated/strangulated hernia	
Prevention	Alcohol screening and brief interventions (see 3.14)	
	Screening (e.g. bowel) and surveillance programmes for GI cancer (e.g. Barrett's oesophagus, patients with colitis or family history of cancer)	
	Diet and nutrition advice	
	Obesity and weight management	
	Smoking cessation	
	Vaccination for at-risk patients (e.g. Hep B)	

The condensed skills

		☑ or score (1–5)
Consultation skills	Recognising that some patients find digestive problems, particularly lower GI, difficult to discuss openly and may be embarrassed and reluctant to undergo rectal examination	
	Communicating the effects of psychological stress on the GI tract in a manner the patient can accept	

Continued over

Examination skills	Abdominal examination (including recognition of the acute abdomen, hepatosplenomegaly and abdominal masses)	
	Rectal examination	
	Proctoscopy	

The condensed know-how

	☑ **or score (1–5)**
How to recognise and respond urgently to alarm ('red flag') symptoms, which may indicate serious pathology (such as GI cancer, obstruction or haemorrhage), the indications for urgent referral and the role of rapid-access GI investigations (and how to use them locally). **Tip:** *Familiarise yourself with the local two-week wait pathway for patients with suspected GI malignancies*	
The evidence-based approach to managing dyspepsia, including guidelines, red flags, investigations and the role of endoscopy and prescribing	
Be familiar with the national screening programme for colorectal cancer. **Tip:** *There is a good summary on: www.cancerscreening.nhs.uk/bowel*	
Resourcing issues: the rationale for restricting upper GI endoscopy in the management of benign dyspepsia and the need for increased availability of lower GI endoscopy for the management of colorectal cancer	
Knowing (and minimising) the GI side effects of common medications	
Recognising the impact of social and cultural diversity, and the importance of health beliefs relating to diet, nutrition and GI function. **Tip:** *The British Nutrition Foundation (www.nutrition.org.uk) offers advice on cultural diversity and diet*	
Key national guidelines in the area of digestive problems	

The condensed resources

- NICE clinical guidelines relevant to this section include *Coeliac Disease, Dyspepsia, Faecal Incontinence* and *Irritable Bowel Syndrome*. Available at: http://guidance.nice.org.uk/CG/ Published.

- SIGN guidelines relevant to this section include *Diagnosis and Management of Colorectal Cancer, Dyspepsia* and *Management of Hepatitis C*. Available at: www.sign.ac.uk/guidelines.

- The RCGP has produced an online course for GPs on diagnosing pancreatic cancer: www.elearning.rcgp.org.uk.

- Specific web resources:

  o Primary Care Society for Gastroenterology: www.pcsg.org.uk

  o British Society of Gastroenterology: www.bsg.org.uk.

Statement 3.14: *Care of People Who Misuse Drugs and Alcohol*

All GPs have a responsibility for providing general medical care to patients who use alcohol and drugs. GPs can help to identify, and intervene in, misuse before it becomes problematic, reducing harm and improving wellbeing for these patients and for their children and families. Both alcohol and drug misuse is amenable to treatment, using a combination of psychological, social and medical interventions. Substitution treatment (such as methadone), if properly administered, results in improvements in social, medical and psychological functioning, and a reduction in criminal behaviour.

GPs must be familiar with ways of identifying and responding to excess alcohol consumption. Despite the prevalence of patients presenting with problems relating to excessive alcohol intake, doctors often fail to make the association. GPs should be aware of the morbidity (physical, psychological and social) caused by alcohol and become practised in a technique called 'brief intervention' (see below), which can have a major impact in reducing alcohol consumption in patients.

The condensed knowledge

		☑ or score (1–5)
Symptoms	Opiate misuse (needle tracks, pinpoint pupils, runny nose, drowsiness)	
	Physical manifestations of alcohol and drug problems (accidents, violence, obesity, dyspepsia, erectile dysfunction, fits, foetal alcohol syndrome, blood-borne infections, liver damage, anaemia, neurological damage)	
	Psychological manifestations of alcohol and drug problems (anxiety, depression, parasuicide)	
	Symptoms of stimulant misuse (agitation, collapse, palpitations, skin ulceration)	
	Symptoms suggestive of cannabis use (red eyes, irritability, anxiety and panic)	

		☑ **or score (1–5)**
Conditions	Complications of drug use and misuse relating to the drugs themselves, routes of use and the associated lifestyle issues	
	Chronic liver disease	
	Hepatitis B and C	
	HIV	
Investigation	Urine (and other) tests for drug treatment	
	Screening tools for alcohol abuse (e.g. CAGE and AUDIT)	
Treatment	Care of drug-abusing patients	
	Safe prescribing for drug-abusing patients	
	Brief interventions for excess alcohol use	
	Management of physical drug and alcohol withdrawal	
Emergencies	Alcohol-related emergencies (e.g. fits, delirium and psychosis)	
	Life-threatening drug-related emergencies (e.g. collapse, coma, overdose)	
	Services available for patients (or families) in crisis	
Prevention	Screening and early intervention strategies in the consultation and the practice for those at risk of alcohol or drug misuse	
	Harm reduction approach	
	Safeguarding for children and vulnerable adults	
	Vaccination of at-risk patients (e.g. Hep B)	

The condensed skills

		☑ or score (1–5)
Consultation skills	Establishing and maintaining rapport with patients with drug and alcohol misuse problems, given the chaotic and challenging ways they may use the health service	
	Opportunistic screening and brief intervention skills to identify and respond to patients at risk of (or engaging in) harmful alcohol use	
	Enabling patients to recognise that a problem exists, engaging them in delineating their difficulties and deciding on appropriate interventions	
Reflective and self-awareness skills	Considering issues around stigma and social exclusion, and awareness of your attitudes to these challenging groups of patients	
Risk assessment skills	Performing drug use assessment and suicide/self-harm risk assessment	
	Mental state assessment (and the difficulties involved in assessing an intoxicated patient)	

The condensed know-how

	☑ or score (1–5)
Recognition that harmful use is often undetected by GPs and can take a range of forms (including binges, excessive use, risk-taking behaviours or dependency)	
The ways patients who use illicit drugs present to services, and the factors that lead to the neglect of health and health care in this group, and steps to counter these.	
Tip: *Review the notes of some of your known drug misusers. Are they receiving optimal physical and mental health care? If not, why not?*	

	☑ **or score** **(1–5)**
The role of the wider primary healthcare team, how to access specialists in secondary care and partnerships with the voluntary and criminal justice sector. **Tip:** *Arrange to spend some time with a community addictions worker*	
The multifactorial causes of drug and alcohol misuse and the relationship with mental health problems	
The relationship between drug misuse and offending behaviour. **Tip:** *Try to arrange some time with a prison doctor, possibly as an attachment or by arranging for him or her to resource a seminar for your learning group*	
The vulnerability of children whose parents are drug users and how to intervene appropriately	
Cultural factors that can mask or complicate alcohol or drug misuse in some communities	
The advice on driving for alcohol and drug users, including the doctor's and the patient's responsibilities	
How the Misuse of Drugs Act 1971 impacts on health professionals treating drug users. **Tip:** *Find out how to prescribe methadone and Subutex, in particular how to arrange for supervised consumption … and what to do if a patient reports that the 'dog ate the prescription'*	
The political changes that impact on the management of drug users	
Ethical issues around adopting a person-centred approach while acknowledging the conflicts between a perceived self-inflicted problem and a right to evidence-based treatment	

The condensed resources

- NICE clinical guidelines relevant to this section include *Alcohol Dependence and Harmful Alcohol Use, Alcohol-Use Disorders: physical complications, Drug Misuse: opioid detoxification, Drug Misuse: psychosocial interventions* and *Psychosis with Coexisting Substance Misuse*. Available at: http://guidance.nice.org.uk/CG/Published.

- NICE Public Health Guidance relevant to this section includes *Alcohol Use Disorders: preventing harmful drinking* and *Needle and Syringe Programmes*.

- The NICE alcohol dependence quality standard is available at: www.nice.org.uk/guidance/qualitystandards/alcoholdependence/home.jsp.

- SIGN guidelines relevant to this section include *The Management of Harmful Drinking and Alcohol Dependence in Primary Care* and *Management of Hepatitis C*. Available at: www.sign.ac.uk/guidelines.

- The RCGP provides a number of online courses for GPs on alcohol- and drug-related health issues (www.elearning.rcgp.org.uk). The e-learning components can be taken independently for self-study or can be combined with a classroom-based workshop to lead to a formal certification:

  ○ 'RCGP harm reduction, health and wellbeing of substance users'

  ○ 'RCGP management of drug misuse in primary care (Parts 1 and 2)'

  ○ 'RCGP management of alcohol problems in primary care'.

- The RCGP Substance Misuse and Associated Health (SMAH) unit is a network of GPs with an interest in improving the health of substance users (www.rcgp.org.uk/substance_misuse.aspx).

- Other web-based resources:

○ the Home Office website has lots of information on national strategies (www.homeoffice.gov.uk/drugs)

○ Talk to Frank offers a handy A–Z of slang names for drugs and other advice for the public on drugs (www.talktofrank.com)

○ The UK Drug Policy Commission (UKDPC) is an independent organisation focusing on the evidence around drug policy and practice (www.ukdpc.org.uk)

○ The National Treatment Agency for Substance Misuse (www.nta.nhs.uk) is an NHS agency working to improve drug treatment services in England.

Brief intervention model: 'FRAMES'[42]

F	Feedback	Assessment and evaluation of the problem
R	Responsibility	Emphasising that drinking is by choice
A	Advice	Explicit advice on changing drinking behaviour
M	Menu	Offering alternative goals and strategies
E	Empathy	The role of the counsellor is important
S	Self-efficacy	Instilling optimism that the chosen goals can be achieved

Statement 3.15: *Care of People with ENT, Oral and Facial Problems*

Ear, nose, and throat (ENT) problems are common reasons for a visit to the GP. Guidelines for appropriate management of ENT problems are widely available but not widely used. Inappropriate referrals to secondary care increase waiting times and consume resources. At the same time, delayed referral of serious conditions can be harmful to patients as early diagnosis and treatment of head and neck cancer is vital. There are around 9 million deaf and hard-of-hearing people in the UK, who face considerable communication barriers. Although some oral conditions are best managed by dentists, these problems commonly present to GPs.

The condensed knowledge

		☑ or score (1–5)
Symptoms	Catarrh, post-nasal drip and nasal obstruction	
	Discharging ear	
	Dizziness	
	Dysphagia	
	Epistaxis	
	Facial pain (e.g. Bell's palsy, temporomandibular pain and trigeminal neuralgia)	
	Facial weakness	
	Hearing loss and tinnitus	
	Hoarseness or voice change	
	Neck swellings (e.g. goitre, lymph nodes and other lumps)	
	Otalgia	
	Sore throat or globus	
	Speech delay	
	Vertigo	

		☑ **or score (1–5)**
Conditions	Croup	
	Ear wax	
	Gingivitis and common dental problems	
	Labyrinthitis, vestibulitis and Ménière's disease	
	Laryngitis and voice strain	
	Nasal polyps	
	Otitis externa	
	Otitis media (suppurative/secretory)	
	Perforated tympanic membrane and cholesteatoma	
	Pharyngitis and tonsillitis; bacterial, viral, glandular fever	
	Rhinitis (infective and allergic)	
	Salivary stones and tumours	
	Sinusitis (infective and allergic)	
	Snoring and sleep apnoea	
	Suspected head and neck cancer	
	Tongue and buccal disorders; oral candidiasis; burning mouth syndrome	
	Trauma (e.g. nasal fracture, haematoma auris)	
	Ulcers or other oral lesions (e.g. aphthous, malignant, oral lichen planus)	
	Unilateral hearing loss (e.g. acoustic neuroma).	
Investigation	Awareness of key specialist investigations (e.g. pure tone threshold audiogram; speech audiometry, impedance tympanometry, auditory brainstem responses and otoacoustic emissions)	
	Awareness that inappropriate investigation may delay referral in suspected head and neck cancer	

Continued over

	☑ or score (1–5)
Treatment Watchful waiting and use of delayed prescriptions for self-limiting conditions	
Long-term treatments for chronic conditions	
Emergencies Auricular haematoma or perichondritis	
Epistaxis	
Foreign bodies (e.g. in ear or nose)	
Fracture of the nose (need manipulation under anaesthetic within two weeks for optimum result)	
Otitis externa (severe); mastoiditis	
Septal haematoma	
Tonsillitis with quinsy	
Prevention Awareness of iatrogenic causes of ototoxicity	
Reducing harmful sound exposure	
Screening for hearing impairment in adults and children	

The condensed skills

	☑ or score (1–5)
Communication skills Communicating effectively with patients with hearing impairment (e.g. remembering to face patients and speaking clearly so that they can lip read)	
Dealing effectively with parental concerns regarding common ENT conditions in children (e.g. glue ear, tonsillitis and otitis media)	
Consultation skills Utilise time as a diagnostic tool (e.g. glue ear), ensuring clear review procedures and safety-netting	

	☑ or score (1–5)
Negotiation skills — To make referrals appropriately and accurately so people with minor ENT conditions do not compromise the care of those with more serious conditions	
Examination skills — Otoscopy	
Simple nasal cautery	
Throat and neck examination	
Tuning-fork tests (Weber and Rinne's tests)	

The condensed know-how

	☑ or score (1–5)
An evidence-based approach to antibiotic prescribing for ENT conditions. **Tip:** *See Cochrane reviews on antibiotic prescribing for common ENT conditions at: www.cochrane.org*	
Symptoms that fall within the range of normal and require no treatment (e.g. cyclical blocking of nose, senile rhinorrhoea, small neck lymph nodes in well children)	
Indications for appropriate referral to an ENT or dental specialist (e.g. recurrent tonsillitis, ear drum perforations in pars flaccida, dental abscess) and the local routes to access these	
Issues arising when services are deficient or have long waiting times for ENT surgery (e.g. audiometry, hearing aids, cochlear implants) and alternatives to specialist referral (e.g. direct-access hearing aid services, email advice services, general practitioner with a special interest [GPwSI], nurse-led clinics, etc.) **Tip:** *What routes of referral can you offer patients in your area who want to be considered for a hearing aid?*	
The role of specialist ENT nurse services and how to access these. **Tip:** *Find out if your local ENT nurses offer urgent aural toilet for more severe cases of otitis externa*	

Continued over

	☑ **or score** **(1–5)**
The role of self-treatment and how to encourage self-coping strategies where appropriate (e.g. hay fever, nosebleeds, dizziness, tinnitus).	
The alarm ('red flag') symptoms for head and neck cancer (e.g. hoarseness persisting for more than six weeks, ulceration of oral mucosa persisting for more than three weeks). **Tip:** *Review the NICE guideline on referral for suspected cancer and review the 'red-flag' symptoms and signs*	
The ENT presentations of systemic or non-ENT diseases, e.g. GORD, CVA, AIDS	
The national screening programme for detecting hearing loss in neonates. **Tip:** *Find out about the Newborn Hearing Screening Programme at: http://hearing.screening.nhs.uk/*	
How certain ENT symptoms can indicate psychological distress (e.g. globus – sensation of not swallowing in a patient who can swallow, the 'dizzy' patient who can walk without difficulty)	
The impact of deafness on people's lives and methods to address this, and ways of ensuring that a patient's hearing impairment does not prejudice the communicated information (e.g. using hearing aid loop induction). **Tip:** *Action on Hearing Loss (www.actiononhearingloss.org.uk) offers advice and support in this area*	
The cultural and social aspects of ENT conditions (e.g. smoking tobacco, cannabis or chewing tobacco, paan, betel nut, khat/qat) and the impact of these on risk assessment and lifestyle advice	
How to provide communications support, such as a BSL/English interpreter or purchasing helpful equipment and putting a prominent reminder on the medical records to alert staff. **Tip:** *What strategies does your practice use to ensure patients with hearing impairment are not disadvantaged?*	
The legal implications of the Equality Act 2010 for GPs including the need for 'reasonable adjustments' for people with hearing impairment (e.g. allowing more time for appointments)	

	☑ **or score**
	(1–5)
The key national guidelines that influence healthcare provision for ENT problems	

The condensed resources

- NICE clinical guidelines relevant to this section include *Respiratory Tract Infections* and *Surgical Management of OME*. Available at: http://guidance.nice.org.uk/CG/Published.

- SIGN guidelines relevant to this section include *Diagnosis and Management of Head and Neck Cancer, Diagnosis and Management of Childhood Otitis Media in Primary Care* and *Management of Sore Throat and Indications for Tonsillectomy*. Available at: www.sign.ac.uk/guidelines.

- The ENT UK website from the British Association of Otorhinolaryngologists, Head and Neck Surgeons contains information and resources on many ENT conditions (www.entuk.org).

Statement 3.16: *Care of People with Eye Problems*

Around 2 million people in the UK have a sight problem, around 1 million of whom are blind or partially sighted. Eye problems account for 1.5% of GP consultations in the UK with a rate of 50 consultations per 1000 population per year. Eye problems are a significant cause of preventable disabilities and the primary healthcare team plays a key role in the prevention and treatment of eye problems.

The condensed knowledge

		☑ or score (1–5)
Symptoms	Altered vision (e.g. flashes, floaters, distortions, halos)	
	Diplopia and strabismus	
	Sticky or itchy eyes	
	Sudden loss of vision (partial or complete)	
	The painful eye	
	The red eye	
Conditions	*Disorders of the lids and lacrimal drainage apparatus:*	
	Blepharitis	
	Stye and chalazion	
	Entropion and ectropion	
	Naso-lacrimal obstruction and dacryocystitis	
	External eye conditions:	
	Conjunctivitis (infective and allergic)	
	Dry-eye syndrome	
	Episcleritis and scleritis	
	Corneal ulcers and keratitis	
	Iritis and uveitis	
	Orbital cellulitis	

		☑ **or score** **(1–5)**
Conditions	*Disorders of refraction:*	
	Cataract	
	Myopia, hypermetropia, astigmatism	
	Principles of refractive surgery	
	Problems associated with contact lenses	
	Disorders of aqueous drainage:	
	Acute angle closure glaucoma	
	Primary open angle glaucoma	
	Secondary glaucomas	
	Vitreo-retinal disorders:	
	Flashes and floaters	
	Macular degeneration	
	Retinal detachment	
	Retinoblastoma	
	Vitreous detachment	
	Vitreous haemorrhage	
	Disorders of the optic disc and visual pathways:	
	Swollen optic disc: recognition and differential diagnosis	
	Atrophic optic disc: recognition and differential diagnosis	
	Pathological cupping of the optic disc	
Investigation	Understanding of appropriate investigations for systemic disease (e.g. erythrocyte sedimentation rate [ESR] for temporal arteritis, chest X-ray [CXR] for sarcoid, etc.)	
	Knowledge of secondary care investigations and treatment including slit lamp and eye pressure measurement	

Continued over

		☑ or score (1–5)
Treatment	Medications including mydriatics, topical anaesthetics, corticosteroids, antibiotics, glaucoma agents	
Emergencies **Tip:** *Find out how to access emergency eye services in your locality*	Superficial ocular trauma, including assessment and management of foreign bodies, abrasions and minor lid lacerations	
	Arc eye	
	Chemical burns	
	Severe injury, including immediate management of penetrating ocular injury, blow-out fracture and hyphaema	
	Retained intra-ocular foreign body	
	Sudden painless loss of vision (e.g. retinal detachment)	
	Severe ocular and peri-ocular infection	
	Acute angle closure glaucoma	
Prevention	Genetics – family history	
	Co-morbidities, especially diabetes and hypertension	

The condensed skills

		☑ or score (1–5)
Consultation skills	Communicating effectively and sensitively with patients with visual impairment and with their carers	
Procedures	Measurement of visual acuity and pinhole testing	
	External examination of the eye and eversion of eyelid	
	Examination of pupil and assessment of red reflex	
	Assessment of ocular movements and cover testing	
	Visual field testing by confrontation	
	Direct ophthalmoscopy	
	Colour vision testing	
	Fluorescein staining of the cornea	

The condensed know-how

	☑ or score (1–5)
Managing ocular manifestations of neurological disease (e.g. hemianopia, nystagmus, manifestations of pituitary and cerebral tumours)	
Managing ocular manifestations of systemic disease (e.g. diabetic retinopathies, retinal vascular occlusions, amaurosis fugax/transient ischaemic attacks [TIAs], hypertensive retinopathy)	
The organisation of screening for eye problems, how to identify those at risk and how to access services (e.g. screening for diabetic retinopathy, glaucoma, visual acuity testing, squint, etc.) **Tip:** *Find out where to direct diabetic patients in need of retinal screening and review the criteria for who should have glaucoma screening*	
When and how to register a patient for blindness and partial sightedness, the value of registration and the role of specialist social workers. **Tip:** *Find out the criteria for registration as blind and the procedure for how a patient registers*	
The psychological and social problems associated with adjustment to chronic visual impairment on the patient, carers and family **Tip:** *Arrange for a visually impaired person to talk to your learning group about his or her experience of daily living*	
The impact of eye problems on disability and fitness to work, the long-term care needs of patients with debilitating eye conditions and the necessary environmental adaptations and use of community resources	
Strategies to help a patient maximise visual function through management of disease, preventive care and control of environmental factors, and how to facilitate patient access to sources of support, including:	
● Royal National Institute of Blind People (RNIB) talking book and return to work services	
● social services; care of the family and financial support	
● local services	
● low-vision aids	
Sources of social and educational support for the visually impaired child. **Tip:** *The National Blind Children's Society website is a good place to start finding out about this: www.nbcs.org.uk*	

Continued over

	☑ **or score (1–5)**
The role of the community optician and appropriate indications for referral	
The role of other primary care health professionals, optometrists, ophthalmologists, orthoptists, school health services, community eye clinics, and social workers in the care of people with eye problems. **Tip:** *Arrange a session in your local eye casualty clinic*	
The DVLA driving regulations for people with visual problems. **Tip:** *These can be found at: www.dft.gov.uk/dvla/medical/ataglance.aspx*	
Strategies for managing the communication issues arising from visual impairment in daily life, such as difficulties receiving written information and accessing services	
The key national guidelines that influence healthcare provision for eye problems	
Ethical issues around balancing the autonomy of patients with visual problems and public safety (e.g. driving)	

The condensed resources

- Royal National Institute of Blind People: www.rnib.org.uk.

- Royal College of Ophthalmologists: www.rcophth.ac.uk.

- NICE has provided guidance on *Glaucoma* and *Type 2 Diabetes – retinopathy*. Available at: http://guidance.nice.org.uk/CG/ Published.

- *e*-GP contains RCGP e-learning sessions on eye problems, covering the key topics in this curriculum statement: www.e-GP.org.

- UK Vision Strategy: www.vision2020uk.org.uk/ UKVisionstrategy.

Statement 3.17: *Care of People with Metabolic Problems*

The prevalence of obesity and diabetes mellitus is increasing, and these conditions are significant risk factors for medical problems. The management of diabetes, hyperthyroidism and hypothyroidism is primarily carried out in primary care and GPs should be competent in the management of diabetic, thyroid and adrenal emergencies. Hyperuricaemia (gout) is a common cause of morbidity, which is usually diagnosed and managed exclusively in primary care.

The condensed knowledge

		☑ or score (1–5)
Symptoms	Patients with metabolic problems are frequently asymptomatic or have non-specific symptoms, such as tiredness, malaise, weight loss or gain	
	Diabetes mellitus – tiredness, polydipsia, polyuria, weight loss, infections	
	Hyperlipidaemia – xanthelasma	
	Hyperuricaemia – gout	
	Hypothyroidism – tiredness, weight gain, constipation, hoarse voice, dry skin and hair, menorrhagia	
	Hyperthyroidism – weight loss, tremor, palpitations, hyperactivity, exophthalmos, double vision	
	Individual endocrine disorders have typical symptom complexes (e.g. polycystic ovary syndrome [PCOS])	
Conditions	Adrenal disease (e.g. Cushing's syndrome, hyperaldosteronism, Addison's disease, phaeochromocytoma)	
	Diabetes mellitus – Type 1 and 2	
	Hyperlipidaemia	
	Hyperuricaemia	
	Impaired Glucose Tolerance (and metabolic syndrome)	

Continued over

		☑ or score (1–5)
Conditions	Obesity	
	Parathyroid disease	
	Pituitary disease (e.g. prolactinoma, acromegaly, diabetes insipidus)	
	Thyroid disorders – hypothyroidism, hyperthyroidism, goitre, thyroid nodules	
Investigation	Body mass index calculation	
	Diagnostic criteria for diabetes mellitus	
	Near-patient capillary glucose measurement (including patient self-monitoring)	
	HbA1c to assess glycaemic control	
	Albumin:creatinine ratio or dipstick for microalbuminuria	
	Interpret serum electrolyte and urate results	
	Interpret thyroid function tests and understand their limitations – TSH, T4, free T4, T3, autoantibodies	
	Interpret lipid profile tests – total cholesterol, HDL, LDL, triglycerides	
	Visual acuity testing and retinal photography	
	Knowledge of secondary care investigations including the glucose tolerance test, thyroid ultrasound and fine needle aspiration, specialised endocrine tests	
Treatment	Understand principles of treatment for common conditions managed largely in primary care – obesity, diabetes mellitus, hypothyroidism, hyperlipidaemia, hyperuricaemia	
	Chronic disease management including specific disease management, systems of care and multidisciplinary teamwork for people with established metabolic problems	
	Communication with patients and their families and inter-professional communication both within the primary healthcare team and between primary and secondary care	

		☑ or score (1–5)
Emergencies	Acute management of diabetic emergencies – hypoglycaemia, hyperglycaemic ketoacidosis and hyperglycaemic hyperosmolar non-ketotic coma	
	Acute management of thyroid emergencies (e.g. hyperthyroid crisis)	
	Recognition and immediate and ongoing management of Addisonian crisis	
Prevention	Health promotion activities include dietary modification and exercise advice	
	Understand when prevention of hyperuricaemia is appropriate, e.g. patients with recurrent gout	
	Obesity and diabetes mellitus are risk factors for other conditions, so optimal management is preventive	

The condensed skills

		☑ or score (1–5)
Consultation skills	Promoting lifestyle change while ensuring that a patient's condition does not prejudice the information communicated and that the risks of complications are not misleadingly stated (e.g. to coerce a patient)	
	Supporting self-care and encouraging concordance with treatment	
Procedures	Calculating body mass index	
	Lower-leg examination for complications of diabetes mellitus	
	Capillary glucose measurement using a near-patient test	
	Thyroid examination	

The condensed know-how

	☑ or score (1–5)
Environmental and genetic factors affecting the prevalence of metabolic problems, diabetes, hypertension and dyslipidaemia. **Tip:** *Diabetes is more prevalent in the UK in patients of Asian and Afro-Caribbean origin, and hyperuricaemia is more prevalent in prosperous areas and is associated with obesity*	
The local systems of care for metabolic conditions, including the roles of primary and secondary care, shared-care arrangements, multidisciplinary teams and patient involvement	
The role of other primary care health professionals, such as diabetes nurse specialists, dieticians, district nurses, community matrons, chiropodists and opticians in chronic disease management. **Tip:** *Find out how to refer patients to the local diabetes specialist nurses, dieticians and podiatrists*	
The indications for referral to an endocrinologist or diabetologist for management of complex metabolic problems or investigation of certain endocrine disorders (e.g. hyperthyroidism)	
Risk factors and the role of screening and recognising symptom complexes, as patients with metabolic problems are frequently asymptomatic or have non-specific symptoms. **Tip:** *What screening does your practice offer to patients at risk of developing Type 2 diabetes? Who should be screened and how do you reach them?*	
Evidence-based lifestyle interventions for obesity, diabetes mellitus, hyperlipidaemia and hyperuricaemia, and the GP's role in promoting and supporting these in the consultation and in the practice. **Tip:** *Arrange an attachment with the community dietician*	
Medications used in the management of diabetes (e.g. glucose-lowering agents, antiplatelet drugs, angiotensin-converting enzyme inhibitors, angiotensin-II receptor antagonists, and lipid-lowering therapies). **Tip:** *What is the latest evidence on the role of aspirin for primary prevention in patients with diabetes?*	
The issues raised by co-morbidity and polypharmacy in diabetes, and strategies to simplify medication regimes and encourage concordance	

	☑ **or score** **(1–5)**
Exemptions from prescription charges for patients with metabolic and endocrine conditions. **Tip:** *Familiarise yourself with FP92A (Medical Exemption Certificate)*	
How to recognise and respond to the psychosocial impact of diabetes and other long-term metabolic problems (e.g. risk of depression, restrictions on employment and driving for diabetes, sexual dysfunction), and the stigma associated with obesity. **Tip:** *Find out about the evidence for ways of screening for depression in chronic disease*[32]	
How to encourage self-management of metabolic conditions and the role of expert patients	
The key national guidelines that influence healthcare provision for cardiovascular problems (e.g. NICE guidelines, British Hypertension Society Joint Committee Recommendations, NSFs and NICE quality standards) and the key research findings that influence management of metabolic problems. **Tip:** *The NICE quality standard for diabetes in adults is available at: www.nice.org.uk/guidance/qualitystandards/diabetesinadults/ diabetesinadultsqualitystandard.jsp. A summary of the NSF for diabetes can be found at: www.nhs.uk/NHSEngland/NSF/Pages/Diabetes.aspx*	

The condensed resources

- NICE clinical guidelines relevant to this section include *Obesity, Type 1 Diabetes, Type 2 Diabetes* and *Type 2 Diabetes – newer agents*. Available at: http://guidance.nice.org.uk/CG/Published.

- SIGN guidelines relevant to this section include *Management of Diabetes* and *Management of Obesity*. Available at: www.sign. ac.uk/guidelines.

- *e*-GP contains RCGP e-learning sessions on metabolic and endocrine problems, covering the key topics in this curriculum statement: www.e-GP.org.

- The full statement has a list of relevant resources in the 'Further reading' section. Two key studies are DCCT (Diabetes Control and Complications Trial) and UKPDS (UK Prospective Diabetes Study).

- The National Obesity Forum is an organisation for professionals interested in obesity: www.nationalobesityforum.org.uk.

- Specific web resources:

  o Association of British Clinical Diabetologists: www.diabetologists-abcd.org.uk

  o Diabetes UK: www.diabetes.org.uk

  o Primary Care Diabetes Society: www.pcdsociety.org.

Statement 3.18: *Care of People with Neurological Problems*

The presentation of a neurological problem may indicate the presence of a disorder confined to a part of the nervous system or may indicate the beginning of a multi-system disease. Symptoms presented to the GP and attributable to a neurological cause may be due to minor self-limiting disease or a more serious problem, so GPs must be able to evaluate the need for any required intervention or referral.

The management of epilepsy and Parkinson's disease in primary care are key areas of general practice and GPs should also be competent in the management of neurological emergencies.

The condensed knowledge

		☑ **or score** **(1–5)**
Symptoms	Abnormal movements and chorea	
	Drowsiness and delirium	
	Headache	
	Loss of consciousness and coma	
	Loss of motor function	
	Memory loss and cognitive impairment	
	Numbness, paraesthesia and sensory disturbance	
	Seizures (complex and partial)	
	Tremor (benign, resting and intention)	
	Vertigo and dizziness (neurological, otological, psychological and cardiovascular causes)	
	Vomiting	
Conditions	Common headache syndromes:	
	● tension headache	
	● migraine and cluster headache	
	● medication-induced headache	

Continued over

		☑ **or score (1–5)**
Conditions	Less common but serious headache syndromes:	
	• raised intracranial pressure, tumours	
	• thunderclap headache (e.g. subarachnoid haemorrhage, enlarging aneurysm or migraine)	
	• temporal arteritis	
	• trigeminal neuralgia	
	Amyotrophic lateral sclerosis	
	Cerebral palsy	
	Epilepsy	
	Essential tremor	
	Genetic conditions (e.g. Huntington's disease, neurofibromatosis)	
	Mononeuropathies including trigeminal neuralgia, Bell's palsy, carpal tunnel syndrome and other nerve entrapments (e.g. ulnar, sciatic and femoral nerves)	
	Multiple sclerosis	
	Neurological causes of vertigo (e.g. stroke, multiple sclerosis, trauma and concussion, acoustic neuroma, brain tumours)	
	Parkinson's disease	
	Polyneuropathies including metabolic causes (diabetes, alcohol, B12 and folate, porphyria, uraemia), infectious causes (e.g. Guillain-Barré, postviral, HIV) and drug-induced neuropathy	
	Speech disorders	
	Stroke (haemorrhage and infarction). **Tip:** *Stroke is also covered in statements 3.05:* Care of Older Adults *and 3.12:* Cardiovascular Health	

	☑ or score (1–5)
Investigation Awareness of indications for secondary care investigations and treatment including electroencephalography (EEG), computerised tomography (CT) and magnetic resonance imaging (MRI), nerve conduction studies	
Treatment Principles of treatment for common conditions managed largely in primary care, including epilepsy, headaches, vertigo, neuropathic pain, mononeuropathies, essential tremor and Parkinson's disease	
The indications for specialist referral for diagnosis or ongoing shared management (e.g. epilepsy, multiple sclerosis, Parkinson's disease)	
Emergencies Acute management of meningitis and meningococcal septicaemia, collapse, loss of consciousness or coma	
Understand indications for urgent referral of people with:	
• stroke / TIA	
• intracranial haemorrhage	
• raised intracranial pressure	
• temporal arteritis	
Prevention Health education and accident prevention advice for people with epilepsy	
Understand avoidance of triggers and prophylaxis for migraine	
Investigation of people with a family history of genetic neurological disease (e.g. berry aneurysm, Huntington's disease)	

The condensed skills

		☑ or score (1–5)
Consultation skills	Communicating prognosis truthfully and sensitively to patients with potentially incurable/disabling neurological conditions	
	Sharing uncertainty when required and managing 'difficult' symptoms with multiple causes (e.g. chronic headache, dizziness, possible multiple sclerosis [MS]). **Tip:** *Discuss strategies for tackling medically unexplained symptoms with your learning group*	
	Enhancing self-care, rehabilitation and return to work for people with long-term neurological conditions and supporting their carers	
Examination skills	Examination of cranial nervous system	
	Examination of peripheral nervous system	
	Visual acuity	
	Visual fields	
	Fundoscopic examination	

The condensed know-how

	☑ or score (1–5)
The functional anatomy of the nervous system as required to aid diagnosis. **Tip:** *This is very relevant to diagnosing common conditions such as carpal tunnel syndrome and sciatica*	
Drug interactions and side effects of epilepsy medications, including contraceptive and pregnancy advice, systems for ensuring regular patient reviews and the issues around concordance. **Tip:** *The higher death rate amongst patients with epilepsy may be related to poor seizure control*	
The current DVLA medical standards of fitness to drive for neurological conditions, in particular epilepsy. **Tip:** *Find these at: www.dft.gov.uk/dvla/medical/ataglance.aspx*	

	☑ **or score** **(1–5)**
The impact neurological conditions may have on an individual's or family's social and economic wellbeing	
The key national guidelines that influence healthcare provision for neurological problems. **Tip:** *Neurological conditions are a focus of the NSF for long-term conditions – see www.nhs.uk/NHSEngland/NSF/Pages/Longtermconditions.aspx*	
Ethical principles involved when treating an adult who lacks capacity to consent (e.g. unconsciousness) or who is unable to communicate (e.g. dysphasia)	

The condensed resources

- NICE clinical guidelines relevant to this section include *Epilepsy, Head Injury, Multiple Sclerosis, Neuropathic Pain, Parkinson's Disease, Stroke* and *Transient Loss of Consciousness*. Available at: http://guidance.nice.org.uk/CG/Published.

- The NICE quality standard for *Stroke* is available at: www.nice.org.uk/guidance/qualitystandards/stroke/strokequalitystandard.jsp.

- SIGN guidelines relevant to this section include *Management of Patients with Stroke or TIA, Diagnosis and Pharmacological Management of Parkinson's Disease, Early Management of Patients with a Head Injury, Diagnosis and Management of Headache in Adults* and *Diagnosis and Management of Epilepsy in Adults*. Available at: www.sign.ac.uk/guidelines.

- RCP National Clinical Guidelines for Stroke: www.rcplondon.ac.uk/resources/stroke-guidelines.

- British Association for the Study of Headache: www.bash.org.uk.

- Information about the National Stroke Strategy is available at: www.nhs.uk/NHSEngland/NSF/Pages/Nationalstrokestrategy.aspx.

Statement 3.19: *Respiratory Health*

Respiratory problems, including infections of the upper and lower respiratory tracts, are the most common reason for a consultation in general practice and for emergency medical admission to hospital. There is little evidence to support antibiotic prescribing for most everyday upper respiratory infections and antibiotics should be used appropriately to limit the development of antimicrobial resistance.

Serious respiratory diseases kill one in four people in the UK, and smoking cessation advice is an essential part of health promotion in primary care. The management of asthma and COPD and the encouragement of self-care are key competencies for GPs, and the full involvement of patients in the management of their respiratory problems is essential.

The condensed knowledge

		☑ or score (1–5)
Symptoms	Breathlessness	
	Chest pain	
	Cough	
	Haemoptysis	
	Wheeze	
	Sputum production	
Conditions	Allergy and anaphylaxis	
	Aspiration of a foreign body	
	Asthma	
	Bronchiolitis	
	Bronchitis	
	Chronic cough	
	Chronic interstitial lung diseases	
	Chronic obstructive pulmonary disease (COPD)	

		☑ or score (1–5)
Conditions	Cystic fibrosis	
	Epiglottitis, laryngitis and tracheitis	
	Hypersensitivity pneumonitis	
	Influenza	
	Lung cancer	
	Pneumonia (of any cause)	
	Pneumothorax	
	Pulmonary embolus	
	Sore throats and colds	
	Tonsillitis and peritonsillar abscess	
	Tuberculosis	
Investigation	Serial peak flow measurement, including patient diaries	
	Reversibility testing using peak flow meter	
	Spirometry	
	Knowledge of secondary care investigations and treatment including lung function tests, computerised tomography (CT) and magnetic resonance imaging (MRI)	
Treatment	Understand principles of treatment for common conditions managed largely in primary care – upper and lower respiratory tract infections, asthma, COPD, allergic reactions and anaphylaxis	
	Inhaler technique for commonly used devices	
Emergency **Tip:** *Learn how to use a nebuliser before an emergency!*	Acute management of people presenting with shortness of breath	
	Management of exacerbations of asthma and COPD	
	Understand indications for emergency referral of people with asthma, COPD and anaphylaxis	

Continued over

		☑ or score (1–5)
Prevention	Smoking cessation assessment, advice and management	
	Vaccination against influenza, Streptococcus pneumoniae, haemophilus influenza B, diphtheria and pertussis	
	Health education advice and patient self-management plans for people with asthma and COPD	
	Understand avoidance of triggers and prophylaxis for allergic conditions	
	Investigation of people with family history of genetic respiratory disease, e.g. cystic fibrosis	

The condensed skills

		☑ or score (1–5)
Consultation skills	Negotiating a self-management plan for asthma in partnership with the patient and sensitively informing patients with incurable or disabling respiratory conditions of their prognosis	
Counselling skills	Giving effective smoking cessation advice and ensuring the doctor–patient relationship is enhanced by this process	
IM&T skills	Using disease registers and data-recording templates effectively for opportunistic and planned monitoring of respiratory problems, and to ensure continuity of care	
Procedures	Peak flow measurement technique using child and adult meters, and accurately interpreting the results	
	Demonstrating and assessing technique for using common inhaler types	
	Performing spirometry and interpreting the results	

The condensed know-how

	☑ **or score**
	(1–5)

The key role of self-care in common self-limiting respiratory conditions (URTI, asthma) and long-term conditions (asthma, COPD).

Tip: *The Asthma UK website contains excellent patient information: www.asthma.org.uk*

_____

An evidence-based approach to antibiotic prescribing for respiratory infections

_____

The causes of breathlessness, including coexisting causes (e.g. simultaneous cardiac and respiratory disease) and optimum management for these

_____

The uses and limitations of serial peak flow measurement, reversibility testing and spirometry in the diagnosis of asthma and COPD.

Tip: *Consider which patients should be screened for COPD (e.g. smoking history, industrial exposure)*

_____

Guidelines for the emergency management and admission of patients with an acute exacerbation of asthma.

Tip: *A brief summary of these can be found in the BNF at the start of the 'Respiratory System' section*

_____

The alarm symptoms for lung cancer and indications for urgent investigation and referral to specialist services.

Tip: *Review the NICE guidelines on referral for suspected cancer (www.nice.org.uk)*

_____

The role of other primary care health professionals, such as practice nurses, district nurses and physiotherapists, in chronic respiratory disease management and pulmonary rehabilitation

_____

Indications for home oxygen therapy and nebulisers, how to evaluate patients' requirements for these, and safety issues when prescribing home oxygen.

Tip: *Find out about the practicalities of prescribing and delivering home oxygen and completing a 'HOOF' (Home Oxygen Order Form) at: www.homeoxygen.nhs.uk*

_____

Common patient health beliefs regarding smoking and ways to reinforce, modify or challenge these beliefs as appropriate

_____

Continued over

	☑ **or score** **(1–5)**
The prevalence of respiratory problems in the community and the current population trends in the prevalence of allergic and respiratory conditions, and particular groups of patients at higher risk of acquiring a respiratory infection	
Occupational exposure as a cause of respiratory disease (e.g. COPD)	
Disability suffered by people with chronic respiratory problems and its psychosocial impact on the patient, family and society. **Tip:** *Look into the local pulmonary rehabilitation service*	
How a GP's personal opinion regarding smoking may influence management decisions for people with respiratory problems	
The key national guidelines that influence healthcare provision for respiratory problems. **Tip:** *An overview of the national strategy for COPD is available at: www. nhs.uk/NHSEngland/NSF/Pages/ChronicObstructivePulmonaryDisease.aspx*	

The condensed resources

- NICE clinical guidelines relevant to this section include *Chronic Obstructive Pulmonary Disease, Lung Cancer* and *Respiratory Tract Infections*. Available at: http://guidance.nice.org.uk/CG/ Published.

- The NICE COPD quality standard is available at: www.nice.org.uk/guidance/qualitystandards/ chronicobstructivepulmonarydisease/copdqualitystandard.jsp.

- SIGN guidelines relevant to this section include *Asthma* (joint with BTS), *Bronchiolitis in Children, Management of Obstructive Sleep Apnoea/Hypopnoea Syndrome in Adults* and *Community Management of Lower Respiratory Tract Infection in Adults*. Available at: www.sign.ac.uk/guidelines.

- The British Thoracic Society (www.brit-thoracic.org.uk) has lots of guidelines pertinent to primary care, including asthma (joint with SIGN), COPD, cough, lung cancer, pneumonia, suspected pulmonary embolism, pulmonary rehabilitation, sleep apnoea and smoking cessation.

- The Primary Care Respiratory Society UK is an organisation for primary care practitioners with a special interest in chest medicine: www.pcrs-uk.org.

- The RCGP's online course 'Respiratory health' contains e-learning sessions covering the key topics in this curriculum statement (www.elearning.rcgp.org.uk).

- Specific web-based resources:

  ○ Asthma UK: www.asthma.org.uk

  ○ British Lung Foundation: www.lunguk.org

  ○ Education for Health: www.educationforhealth.org.

Statement 3.20: *Care of People with Musculoskeletal Conditions*

Musculoskeletal conditions are common, accounting for around one in four GP consultations. They lead to significant disability and have huge resource implications from causing incapacity to work. The ability to support patients in self-management is of central importance to this area of general practice.

The condensed knowledge

		☑ or score (1–5)
Symptoms	Inflammation – pain, swelling, redness, warmth	
	Injuries – cuts, bruises, burns, wounds, sprains, fractures	
	Loss of function – weakness, restricted movement, deformity and disability	
	Alarm symptoms ('red flags') suggestive of infection, fracture, inflammatory arthritis, malignancy or neurological compromise requiring prompt or immediate referral	
	Common patterns of symptoms and signs in children, including normal variants, potentially serious conditions and possible non-accidental injury	
	Systemic manifestations of musculoskeletal disease – rashes, tiredness, weight loss, etc.	
Conditions in adults	Acute arthropathies	
	Back/neck pain – acute	
	Back/neck pain – chronic	
	Chronic disability	
	Chronic inflammatory arthropathies	
	Common injuries and sprains	

	☑ **or score (1–5)**
Conditions in adults Fibromyalgia and allied syndromes	
Fractures	
Head injury	
Internal injuries of the chest, abdomen and pelvis	
Knee pain (e.g. ligamentous injuries, cartilage tears, arthritis)	
Osteoarthritis	
Osteoporosis.	
Tip: *Online calculators for fracture risk in osteoporosis include FRAX (www.shef.ac.uk/FRAX) and QFracture (www.qfracture.org)*	
Pain management (including regional pain syndromes and multiple-site pain)	
Polymyalgia rheumatica and related conditions	
Shoulder disorders (e.g. rotator cuff tears, capsulitis, impingement)	
Soft-tissue disorders (e.g. bursitis, synovitis, tendonitis)	
Awareness of less common musculoskeletal and rheumatological conditions requiring prompt or immediate referral (e.g. septic arthritis, osteomyelitis, bony metastases, sarcoma, pathological fracture, cauda equina syndrome)	

Continued over

		☑ **or score (1–5)**
Conditions in children	Knowledge of conditions in children and the typical ages when they present, including:	
	● anterior knee pain	_____
	● developmental dysplasia of the hip	_____
	● hypermobility	_____
	● juvenile idiopathic arthritis	_____
	● Perthe's disease	_____
	● rickets	_____
	● scoliosis	_____
	● septic arthritis	_____
	● slipped upper femoral epiphysis	_____
	● subluxation of the radial head ('pulled elbow')	_____
	● traction apophysitis (Osgood–Schlatter and Sever's disease)	_____
Investigation	Indications for plain radiography, ultrasound, CT and MRI including the use of tools such as the 'Ottawa Rules'	_____
	General principles of X-ray indications, interpretation and common errors	_____
	Indications for blood investigations in diagnosis and management, and their limitations in diagnosis	_____
Treatment	Understand the evidence-based principles of treatment for common conditions managed largely in primary care (e.g. back pain, osteoarthritis, gout, polymyalgia)	_____
	Knowledge of the use and monitoring of analgesia, NSAIDs, steroids and disease-modifying drugs, and the primary and secondary prevention of adverse effects	_____
	Knowledge of when joint injections and aspirations are appropriate in general practice, and the ability to perform when appropriate, e.g. shoulder and knee joints and injections for tennis and golfer's elbow	_____

	☑ **or score** **(1–5)**

Treatment	Knowledge of indications for orthopaedic referral, including:	
	• back pain with significant nerve root compression or spinal stenosis	
	• meniscal tear or knee ligament injuries	
	• traumatic rotator cuff tear or shoulder subluxation/ dislocation	
	• Achilles tendon rupture	
	Understand the roles of allied health professionals (nursing, physiotherapy, chiropody, podiatry, occupational therapy, counselling and psychological services)	
	Chronic disease management including systems of care, multidisciplinary teamwork and shared-care arrangements. **Tip:** *Audit the regular monitoring of blood tests of patients taking disease-modifying drugs (DMARDs) – known as 'near-patient testing'*	
Emergency	The initial management of the patient who has been burnt	
	To be aware of the safety of the patient, the scene of the incident and medical staff	
	To be aware of how to summon help in an emergency	
	Be competent in reducing pain by the use of analgesia or other methods	
	Be aware of the principles of major incident management	
	Referrals requiring emergency action to save life or prevent serious long-term sequelae	
Prevention	Advice regarding appropriate levels of exercise	
	Heath promotion regarding accident prevention	

Continued over

The condensed skills

		☑ or score (1–5)
Consultation skills	Giving health information positively and effectively to patients and communicating truthfully and sensitively to those for whom therapeutic options are limited	
	Exploring and addressing beliefs that might be preventing recovery (e.g. a perceived incompatibility with work and other activities), shared goal-setting and planning to reduce pain and disability	
	Promoting activity and supporting self-care in accordance with the patient's conditions and abilities	
	Avoiding investigations or treatments unlikely to alter outcomes (e.g. inappropriate back imaging) and prioritising referrals appropriately	
Examination skills	Targeted examination of the following areas:	
	• the neck and back	
	• the shoulder, elbow, wrist and hand	
	• the hip, knee and ankle	
	• Generalised mobility, stiffness, skin changes	

The condensed know-how

	☑ or score (1–5)
The epidemiology of musculoskeletal disorders at all ages, and how this informs a differential diagnosis	
The natural history of common and important musculoskeletal conditions over time and how this pattern informs diagnosis and treatment	
Awareness of the roles of the primary healthcare team, allied health professionals, complementary therapists and secondary care (e.g. in shared-care protocols), and how to refer appropriately to the most appropriate healthcare practitioner (e.g. GPwSI, physiotherapist, podiatrist, osteopath, chiropractor, orthopaedic surgeon and rheumatologist), shared-care arrangements, multidisciplinary teams and expert-patient involvement. **Tip:** *Spend time shadowing a variety of these practitioners*	
How the mechanism of an injury may inform the diagnosis	
How to distinguish inflammatory from non-inflammatory conditions	
Assessment and management of the psychological factors causing or contributing to musculoskeletal symptoms and the concept of 'yellow flags' that indicate a poorer prognosis	
Iatrogenic problems caused by the treatment of musculoskeletal disorders (e.g. GI bleeds, osteoporosis, coronary heart disease) and the prevention of these. **Tip:** *Find out what systems your practice has in place to reduce methotrexate prescribing errors*	
The GP's wider role in the assessment of musculoskeletal disability and mobility. **Tip:** *Find out how patients apply for a disabled parking badge and the GP's role in the process*	
How to access patient educational resources, information leaflets and support groups. **Tip:** *Available at the Arthritis Research UK website: www.arthritisresearchuk.org*	

Continued over

	☑ **or score**
	(1–5)

Self-help strategies to empower the patient, e.g. self-treatment measures, the expert-patient programme (DH), Challenging Arthritis Programme (Arthritis Care) and local exercise programmes.

Tip: *The expert-patient programme (www.expertpatients.co.uk) and the Self Care Forum (www.selfcareforum.org) help people with long-term conditions to develop the skills and confidence to better manage their condition*

The health and economic consequences of long-term worklessness due to musculoskeletal conditions and the skills to support return to work.

Tip: *The Healthy Working UK website contains information and resources for practitioners on sickness certification and supporting patients in returning to work: www.healthyworkinguk.co.uk*

Indications for referral to complementary medical services, considering that many services have limited NHS availability or are only available privately

The role of occupation in musculoskeletal disease (e.g. repetitive strain injury) and the likely prognosis in relation to the occupation as well as the positive effects of work on health

The key national guidelines for musculoskeletal problems

The condensed resources

- NICE clinical guidelines relevant to this section include *Low Back Pain, Osteoarthritis* and *Rheumatoid Arthritis*. Available at: http://guidance.nice.org.uk/CG/Published.

- SIGN guidelines relevant to this section include *Management of Osteoporosis, Management of Early Rheumatoid Arthritis* and *Diagnosis and Management of Psoriasis and Psoriatic Arthritis in Adults*. Available at: www.sign.ac.uk/guidelines.

- *e*-GP contains RCGP e-learning sessions on musculoskeletal and rheumatological conditions, including demonstrations of targeted examinations (www.e-GP.org).

- The RCGP has produced an online course on 'Musculoskeletal skills': www.elearning.rcgp.org.uk.

- Primary Care Rheumatology Society: www.pcrsociety.org.

- National Osteoporosis Society: www.nos.org.uk.

- Arthritis Research UK offers resources and information for health professionals and patients: www.arthritisresearchuk.org.

- Healthy Working UK website contains information, resources and advice for healthcare practitioners on 'fit notes' and supporting patients returning to work: www.healthyworkinguk.co.uk.

- The Disabled Living Foundation website (www.dlf.org.uk) has a section for health professionals and includes useful advice on disability products and disabled equipment for older and disabled people, their carers and families.

Statement 3.21: *Care of People with Skin Problems*

Approximately a quarter of the population are affected by skin problems, most of whom are managed in primary care. Skin disfigurement causes considerable psychological distress and the effective diagnosis and urgent referral of potential melanomas can save lives.

The condensed knowledge

		☑ or score (1–5)
Symptoms	Alarm symptoms ('red flags') for suspicious lesions	
	Causes of bruising or purpura	
	Causes of hair loss (e.g. alopecia)	
	Itchy lesions and rashes	
	Lesions affecting mucous membranes	
	Nail problems	
	Patterns of common skin problems (e.g. flexural, facial)	
	Photosensitivity	
	Pigmented skin lesions	
	Rashes in different age groups	
	Weeping, crusting, inflammation	
Conditions	Acne vulgaris	
	Benign skin lesions (e.g. actinic keratosis, dermatofibroma, lipoma, naevus, seborrhoeic keratosis, skin tag)	
	Common congenital lesions	
	Drug eruptions	
	Eczema	
	Generalised pruritus	
	Genital lesions and rashes	

		☑ **or score** (1–5)
Conditions	Gestational dermatoses	
	Hair and nail disorders	
	Infections of the skin (bacterial, viral and fungal)	
	Infestations including scabies and head lice	
	Ingrowing toenails	
	Leg ulcers and lymphoedema	
	Malignant skin lesions (e.g. basal cell carcinoma, Bowen's disease, malignant melanoma, squamous cell carcinoma)	
	Psoriasis	
	Rosacea	
	Urticaria	
	Vasculitis	
	Awareness of other less common skin conditions such as the bullous disorders, lichen planus, vitiligo, photosensitivity, pemphigus, pemphigoid, lupus, granuloma annulare and lichen sclerosus	
Investigation	Taking specimens for mycology from skin, hair and nail	
	Basic interpretation of histology reports	
	Investigations for systemic conditions that may cause skin symptoms (e.g. iron deficiency, thyroid disorders, gout)	
	Patch and prick testing indications	
	Skin biopsy indications and interpretations	
Treatment	Commonly used treatments in primary care (including an awareness of appropriate quantities to be prescribed and how to apply them).	
	Tip: *Familiarise yourself with the topical steroids potency ladder in the BNF and the concept of 'fingertip units'*	

Continued over

		☑ or score (1–5)
Treatment	An awareness of indications for and side effects of specialised treatments, such as retinoids, ciclosporin, phototherapy and methotrexate	
	Effects of immunosuppression and increased risk of skin malignancies	
	The indications for curettage, cautery and cryosurgery	
Emergency	Angioedema and anaphylaxis	
	Eczema herpeticum	
	Erythroderma	
	Necrotising fasciitis	
	Stevens–Johnson syndrome	
	Toxic epidermal necrolysis	
Prevention	Principles of protective care (sun care, occupational health and hand care)	
	Fixed factors: family history and genetics (how genetic factors influence the inheritance of common diseases such as psoriasis and atopic eczema)	
	Occupation and care of the hands	

The condensed skills

		☑ or score (1–5)
Consultation skills	Eliciting the history of change and evolution of skin problems over time	
	Ensuring that skin problems are not dismissed as trivial and patients with chronic skin problems are helped to manage the effects of disfigurement	
	Assessing risk factors (e.g. in a patient reporting change in a pigmented skin lesion)	

		☑ **or score (1–5)**
Consultation skills	Assessing risk factors (e.g. in a patient reporting change in a pigmented skin lesion)	
	Enabling patients to self-care for common skin problems and to explain the treatments they have already tried	
Examination skills	Performing an adequately exposed but dignified examination of skin, including personal areas	
Procedures	Curettage, cautery and cryosurgery (optional)	
	Specimens for mycology from skin, hair and nail, and use of Wood's light	

The condensed know-how

	☑ **or score (1–5)**
The promotion of skin wellbeing, including sun protection, occupational health advice and hand care, and educating patients about symptoms/signs of potentially serious lesions	
The relevance of family history (e.g. atopy) and contact history (e.g. impetigo, scabies) in some skin conditions	
Criteria for urgent referral to specialist services, especially to rapid-access pathways for suspected malignant lesions	
Alternatives to traditional specialist referral (e.g. email advice services, GPwSI and nurse-led clinics)	
Supporting self-management in skin conditions (e.g. eczema and psoriasis)	
The role of other community-based team members (e.g. district and tissue viability nurses) and shared-care arrangements in the management of many skin problems, e.g. pigmented lesions, leg ulcers, psoriasis	
Common drugs (including over-the-counter meds) that may cause skin problems.	
Tip: *Look up the skin complaints associated with prescribed drugs such as amiodarone, beta-blockers, lithium, steroids (inhaled, systemic and topical), retinoids and tetracyclines*	

Continued over

	☑ **or score (1–5)**
The rationale for restricting certain investigations and treatments in the management of skin problems (e.g. patch testing, prescribing of retinoids, access to phototherapy). **Tip:** *Find out your local referral restrictions for cosmetic skin problems, and consider the difficulties this raises*	
The social and psychological impact of skin problems on quality of life: stigma and the effects of disfigurement, and sleep deprivation as a result of itching. **Tip:** *The Changing Faces charity offers a free simple skin camouflage service. For more information, see www.changingfaces.org.uk*	
Assessing occupational risk (including hobbies) in the aetiology and impact of skin disease	
Guidelines and procedures for ensuring informed consent is obtained for procedures (e.g. minor surgery)	
The key national guidelines that influence healthcare provision for skin problems (e.g. NICE guidance)	

The condensed resources

- NICE clinical guidelines relevant to this section include *Atopic Eczema in Children*. Available at: http://guidance.nice.org.uk/CG/Published.

- SIGN guidelines relevant to this section include *Management of Atopic Eczema in Primary Care, Diagnosis and Management of Psoriasis and Psoriatic Arthritis in Adults* and *Management of Chronic Venous Leg Ulcers*. Available at: www.sign.ac.uk/guidelines.

- British Association of Dermatologists: www.bad.org.uk.

- Primary Care Dermatology Society: www.pcds.org.uk.

- Specific web-based resources:

  ○ DermIS online dermatology atlas: www.dermis.net

  ○ DermNet NZ: www.dermnetnz.org

  ○ Google Images (www.google.co.uk) can be useful for quickly locating pictures of skin conditions, although check the image is an accurate representation and appropriately sourced.

Statement 3.X: *The Rest of General Practice*

The RCGP Curriculum for Specialty Training for General Practice is a competency-based document, describing the core knowledge and skills required to be a GP (as described in Chapter 5, 'The core curriculum'). One of the key competencies a GP must acquire is 'managing primary contact with patients and dealing with unselected problems'. This includes being able to deal with virtually every kind of problem and every kind of patient that walks through the surgery door.

Although the curriculum is a large and comprehensive document, it is inevitable that some clinical topics are not mentioned explicitly. This does not mean such topics should not be learned or taught if appropriate; learning to be a successful GP involves learning whatever needs to be learned to competently perform the role of a generalist physician working in the community.

In this condensed statement, we have included a number of topics that are not explicitly covered by their own curriculum statement. This includes topics that may come up in the MRCGP (see Chapter 4, 'Succeeding at the MRCGP'). GP learners and educators should consider whether they need to incorporate these into their learning and teaching plans when preparing for the MRCGP assessments.

Clinical topics not currently covered by a curriculum statement:

		☑ or score (1–5)
Haematology	Anaemia	
	Bleeding disorders	
	Clotting disorders and VTE/DVT	
	Haematological investigations (e.g. FBC, film, ESR, D-dimers, B12/folate, haematinics)	
	Lymphadenopathy	
	Lymphoproliferative disorders	
	Myelodysplasia and myeloproliferative disorders.	
	Paraproteinaemias and myeloma	

Continued over

		☑ **or score** **(1–5)**
Haematology *(continued)*	Post-splenectomy prophylaxis	
	Red-cell disorders and haemolysis	
	Warfarin (initiation and monitoring)	
Renal problems	Haematuria (and microhaematuria)	
	Glomerulonephritis	
	Nephrotic syndrome	
	Pyelonephritis and UTI	
	Renal function test interpretation and monitoring (e.g. U+E, creatinine, eGFR, 24-hour urinary collection tests, microalbuminaemia, proteinuria, ACR and PCR)	
	Renal impairment and chronic renal failure (CKD has been included in 3.12 *Cardiovascular Health* in this book)	
	Renal and bladder stones	
	Renal tract imaging (e.g. CT, USS)	
	Urinary tract malignancies (e.g. renal, bladder)	
	Tip: *Lower urinary tract problems (e.g. cystitis, urinary incontinence and retention) are covered in the clinical example statements 3.06* Women's Health *and 3.07* Men's Health.	
	Tip: *NICE clinical guidance on CKD is available at: www.nice.org.uk/CG73.*	
	Tip: *the SIGN guideline on CKD is available at: www.sign.ac.uk/guidelines/fulltext/103*	
Infectious diseases	Bacterial infections (e.g. brucellosis, endocarditis, erysipelas staphylococcus, streptococcus, legionella, listeria, Lyme disease, psittacosis, tetanus, treponema)	
	Food poisoning (e.g. botulism, campylobacter, salmonella, *E. coli*, rotavirus)	
	Hospital-acquired infections (e.g. MRSA and clostridium)	

or score
(1–5)

Infectious diseases *(continued)*	Influenza vaccination campaigns and management of high-risk groups; flu pandemic planning	
	Notifiable diseases and role of public health in infectious disease control and contact tracing	
	Parasitic and protozoal infections (e.g. head lice, threadworms, toxoplasmosis, scabies)	
	Postviral fatigue syndrome	
	Pyrexia of unknown origin	
	Routine immunisation schedules and issues around vaccination (e.g. MMR, BCG, pneumovax)	
	Systemic fungal infections (e.g. aspergillosis, oral candidiasis, pityriasis)	
	Travel advice and vaccinations	
	Tropical diseases (malaria, amoebic dysentery, giardiasis), traveller's diarrhoea, malaria prophylaxis	
	Viral infections (e.g. hepatitis A, herpes simplex, herpes zoster, HIV, influenza, infectious mononucleosis, hand, foot and mouth, measles, mumps, parvovirus, rubella)	
Surgery	Evaluating a patient's fitness for surgery	
	Optimising a patient's fitness for surgery	
	Managing common post-surgical complications after discharge	
	Routine wound care and healing	
	Recovery, rehabilitation and return to work after surgery	
Miscellaneous	Medically unexplained symptoms	
	Chronic fatigue	
	Off legs	
	Common occupational health issues	
	Tip: *www.healthyworkinglives.com is a Scottish NHS website with advice on making workplaces healthier and safer*	

Other clinical topics *you* have identified a need to learn

☑ **or score**

(1–5)

References

1 Helman C G. Disease versus illness in general practice. *Journal of the Royal College of General Practitioners* 1981; **31**: 548–62.

2 Rosenstock I. *Historical Origins of the Health Belief Model.* Health Education Monographs. Vol. 2, No. 4, 1974.

3 Pendleton D, Schofield T, Tate P, *et al. The Consultation: an approach to learning and teaching.* Oxford: Oxford University Press, 1984.

4 Caldicott Committee, Department of Health. *Report on the Review of Patient-Identifiable Information.* London: DH, 1997, www.dh.gov.uk [accessed May 2012].

5 Stott N C, Davis R H. The exceptional potential in each primary care consultation. *Journal of the Royal College of General Practitioners* 1979; **29**: 201–5.

6 Neighbour R. *The Inner Consultation.* Lancaster: M T P, 1987.

7 Tuckett D, Boulton M, Olson C, *et al. Meetings between Experts.* London: Tavistock Publications, 1985.

8 Stewart M, Brown J B, Weston W W, *et al.* Patient-centred medicine. In: *Transforming the Clinical Method* (2nd edn). Abingdon: Radcliffe Medical Press, 2003.

9 Kurtz S M, Silverman J D. The Calgary–Cambridge observation guides: an aid to defining the curriculum and organizing the teaching in communication training programmes. *Medical Education* 1996; **30**: 83–9.

10 Kurtz S M, Silverman J D, Draper J. *Teaching and Learning Communication Skills in Medicine*. Oxford: Radcliffe Medical Press, 1998.

11 NHS Institute for Innovation and Improvement. Plan, Do, Study, Act (PDSA). www.institute.nhs.uk/quality_and_service_improvement_tools/quality_and_service_improvement_tools/plan_do_study_act.html [accessed May 2012].

12 National Patient Safety Agency. *Foresight Training Resource Pack 5: examples of James Reason's 'three bucket' model*. London: NPSA, 2008.

13 General Medical Council. *Good Medical Practice*. London: GMC, 2006.

14 Royal College of General Practitioners/General Practitioners Committee. *Good Medical Practice for General Practitioners*. London: RCGP, 2008, www.rcgp.org.uk/pdf/PDS_Good_Medical_Practice_for_GPs_July_2008.pdf [Accessed May 2012].

15 Department of Health (England). *Standards for Better Health*. London: DH, 2004, www.dh.gov.uk/en/Publicationsandstatistics/Publications/PublicationsPolicyAndGuidance/DH_4086665 [Accessed May 2012].

16 Maslow A H. *Motivation and Personality*. New York: Harper & Row, 1954.

17 McClelland D C. *Human Motivation*. San Francisco: Scott Foresman, 1985.

18 Belbin R M. *Management Teams: why they succeed or fail*. Oxford: Butterworth-Heinemann, 1981.

19 www.peterhoney.com [accessed May 2012].

20 Neighbour R. *The Inner Apprentice*. Newbury: Petroc, 1992.

21 Kolb D. *Experiential Learning*. New Jersey: Prentice Hall, 1984.

22 Knowles M. *The Adult Learner: a neglected species* (4th edn). Houston: Gulf Publishing, 1990.

23 Brookfield S D. *Understanding and Facilitating Adult Learning*. San Francisco: Jossey-Bass, 1986.

24 Schön D. *Educating the Reflective Practitioner*. San Francisco: Jossey-Bass, 1987.

25 Heron J. *Helping the Client: a creative practical guide*. London: Sage Publications, 1990.

26 Bolton G. *Reflective Practice: writing and professional development*. London: Paul Chapman Publishing, 2001.

27 Dawes M, Summerskill W, Glasziou P, *et al*. Sicily statement on evidence-based practice. *BMC Medical Education* 2005; **5(1)**: 1.

28 Tudor Hart J. The inverse care law. *Lancet* 1971; **i**: 405–12.

29 Wilson J M G, Junger G. *Principles and Practice of Screening for Disease*. Geneva: WHO, 1968.

30 Hall D, Elliman D. *Health for All Children* (4th edn, revised). Oxford: Oxford University Press, 2006.

31 DiClemente C C, Prochaska J O, Fairhurst S K, *et al*. The process of smoking cessation: an analysis of precontemplation, contemplation, and preparation stages of change. *Journal of Consulting and Clinical Psychology* 1991; **59**: 295–304.

32 Medical Protection Society. *Case Reports* 13(3), August 2005.

33 Department of Health. *Best Practice Guidance for Doctors and Other Health Professionals on the Provision of Advice and Treatment to Young People under 16 on Contraception, Sexual and Reproductive Health*. London: DH, 2004.

34 Fick D M, Cooper J W, Wade W E, *et al*. Updating the Beers criteria for potentially inappropriate medication use in older adults: results of a US consensus panel of experts. *Archives of Internal Medicine* 2003; **163**: 2716–24.

35 Scottish Executive. *Adding Life to Years*. Edinburgh: Scottish Executive, 2002.

36 Cox J L, Holden J M, Sagovsky R. Detection of postnatal depression: development of the 10-item Edinburgh Postnatal Depression Scale. *British Journal of Psychiatry* 1987; **150**: 782–6.

37 R C G P curriculum statement 10.2: *Men's Health*. London: RCGP, 2006.

38 Gillick v West Norfolk and Wisbech Area Health Authority [1986] AC 112, [1985] UKHL 7, [1986] 1 FLR 229.

39 Arroll B, Khin N, Kerse N. Screening for depression in primary care with two verbally asked questions: cross sectional study. *British Medical Journal* 2003; **327**: 1144–6.

40 Heart Protection Study Collaborative Group. M R C / B H F Heart Protection Study of cholesterol lowering with simvastatin in 20,536 high-risk individuals: a randomised placebo-controlled trial. *Lancet* 2002; **360**: 7–22.

41 Drossman D A (Moderator, A G A Clinical Symposium). Rome III: new criteria for the functional G I disorders. In: *Program and abstracts of Digestive Disease Week*, 20–25 May 2006; Los Angeles, California, pp. 461–9.

42 Miller W R, Sanchez V C. Motivating young adults for treatment and lifestyle change. In: G Howard (ed.). *Issues in Alcohol Use and Misuse in Young Adults*. Notre Dame: University of Notre Dame Press, 1993.

Appendix 1
Getting the most from specialty-based placements

The aim of this appendix is to signpost the aspects of the curriculum that are particularly pertinent to the various specialty-based placements that commonly make up the early part of GP training programmes in ST1 and ST2. Of course not all trainees will work in all specialties, and it may not be possible to cover all the things we suggest – but we hope this will be a useful guide to making the most of specialty-based placements.[i]

All GP training placements provide opportunities to hone your clinical and communications skills with patients, families and other healthcare professionals. Most also provide opportunities to work within multidisciplinary teams.

As a general rule in hospital-based specialties, try to maximise your opportunities to attend outpatient clinics – these are full of the types of patients with long-term conditions that you will see most frequently in general practice. If the patient was referred by his or her GP, try to establish why – is the reason for the referral clear in the letter and does it match the expectation of the patient? If not, why do you think that might be? Did the consultant consider the referral appropriate? Were there tests or treatments that perhaps could have been tried prior to referral?

Time on-call/on-take is particularly useful for gaining supervised experience in recognising and managing acutely ill children and adults. Once you are working in general practice, you will need to be able to distinguish these sick patients from the many others with self-limiting illnesses and respond accordingly.

Many specialty-based placements provide great opportunities to learn and document your skills in carrying out specific procedures (e.g. DOPS), although it is important to ensure these are supervised and signed off by an appropriately experienced clinician.

Trainees who find themselves spending an excessive amount of time doing tasks of limited educational value for GP training may find this appendix helpful when trying to negotiate additional educational opportunities with their consultants and other colleagues. It can also be used to develop a plan to maximise the value of short specialty-based attachments.

i The authors are grateful to Dr Helen Ashdown, a GP specialty trainee in the Oxford Deanery, for her help with compiling this appendix.

Placement	Make sure you read	Hints and tips for learning the curriculum
Early general practice placement (in ST1 or 2)	1.0 *Being a General Practitioner*	• A period of experience in general practice is now included early in many GP training programmes (e.g. in ST1). This early experience greatly helps you to understand the holistic, comprehensive, generalist approach required for good general practice. • Gaining some general practice experience early in training is important as it allows you to apply this insight to the activities you undertake in all your subsequent specialty-based placements, making them more effective GP training experiences
Acute general medicine	3.03 *Care of Acutely Ill People* *Also read the relevant clinical example statements (e.g. 3.12 Cardiovascular Health)*	• Hone your skills in assessment and management of common medical emergencies, and in identifying the seriously ill. • Learn about the appropriate use of diagnostic tests and investigations. • Gain experience in managing exacerbations of common illnesses – e.g. COPD or asthma. • Ask senior colleagues to explain the rationale for their decisions on whether or not to admit or discharge particular patients – this will help you in the future when you have to decide whether or not your patient in primary care needs admission to hospital or can be managed safely at home
Dermatology	3.21 *Care of People with Skin Problems*	• Outpatients offer a great opportunity to improve your skills in targeted history taking and symptom pattern recognition, to help you diagnose common skin conditions • Familiarise yourself with the management of common chronic skin conditions – e.g. atopic eczema, contact eczema, psoriasis, pruritus

Placement	Make sure you read	Hints and tips for learning the curriculum
Dermatology *(continued)*	3.21 *Care of People with Skin Problems*	• Learn about the principles of diagnosing and managing undifferentiated rashes. • Gain experience in assessing pigmented and other skin lesions. • Learn from patients about the psychological and social impact of long-term skin conditions and find the sources of support available. • Learn how to use a dermatoscope to examine common skin lesions. • This is a great opportunity to learn and practise minor surgical techniques (e.g. incisions, excisions, biopsies and cryotherapy)
Elderly care	3.05 *Care of Older Adults* *Also read the relevant clinical example statements (e.g. 3.12 Cardiovascular Health)*	• Try to gain a good understanding of the conditions and problems common in older age – e.g. dementia, falls, depression, stroke, Parkinson's disease, acute confusion and general frailty. • Become familiar with locally available services for the elderly – e.g. day hospitals, rapid-access clinics. • Learn about the issues of polypharmacy and how to prescribe safely for older adults. • Find out about medico-legal issues relevant to the elderly (e.g. mental capacity). • Learn about the issues affecting carers, how to involve carers in care-planning, and what support is in place for carers

Continued over

Placement	Make sure you read	Hints and tips for learning the curriculum
Emergency medicine (A&E)	3.03 *Care of Acutely Ill People* *Also read the relevant clinical example statements (e.g. 3.20 Care of People with Musculoskeletal Problems)*	• A&E provides good opportunities to learn about the diagnosis and management of a wide range of common illnesses and ailments – try to understand the deeper reasons why people seek medical help for minor ailments and how you can encourage them to self-care in future. In particular consider what factors influence a person's choice to attend the emergency department when other sources of medical care (e.g. routine GP appointment or 'out of hours' GP) may have been more appropriate. • Gain experience of identifying seriously ill children and adults, and learn how to respond effectively and appropriately to these patients. • Learn how to refer safely and effectively to and work with colleagues, and how to manage and prioritise your workload. • Learn when you should and should not request X-rays and other imaging, especially for limb injuries. This is a good opportunity to learn about the management of other common MSK injuries (e.g. ankles, knees, shoulders and hands). • Become familiar with assessing head injuries and the advice you should provide parents and carers. • Hone your skills in the initial management of life-threatening emergencies – especially anaphylaxis, severe asthma, meningococcal disease, acute coronary syndromes, acute breathlessness, loss of consciousness and cardiac arrest. • Learn how to assess, clean, glue/steristrip/suture and dress minor wounds (including scalds and burns) – this skill will always be useful!

Placement	Make sure you read	Hints and tips for learning the curriculum
End-of-life/ palliative medicine	3.09 *End-of-Life Care*	• Spend time with the Macmillan/end-of-life care nurses.
		• Learn about symptom control in advanced cancer, including pain management.
		• Learn how to recognise the changes that indicate the patient is approaching the final stages of life.
		• Gain experience in holding difficult conversations with patients and their families.
		• Find out about the wider aspects of palliative care including spiritual care, music and art therapy, complementary therapies.
		• Learn how to set up and prescribe safely for a syringe driver.
		• Find out about the legal and administrative issues around death and the after-care available for families.
ENT	3.15 *Care of People with ENT, Oral and Facial Problems*	• Become familiar with the assessment and management of common ENT emergencies – e.g. nosebleeds, tonsillitis, severe otitis externa.
		• This is a good opportunity to learn the specialist management of common ENT conditions seen in primary care – e.g. chronic rhinitis/sinusitis, nasal polyps, glue ear, otitis externa, globus and recurrent tonsillitis.
		• Find out how to diagnose and manage the different causes of facial pain.
		• Learn when to suspect a head and neck malignancy and how to care for people with head and neck cancers.
		• Practise performing and interpreting otoscopy, tuning fork tests, audiometry and tympanometry

Continued over

Placement	Make sure you read	Hints and tips for learning the curriculum
Genito-urinary/ sexual health medicine	3.01 *Healthy People: promoting health and preventing disease* 3.06 *Women's Health* 3.07 *Men's Health* 3.08 *Sexual Health*	• Practise taking a sexual history and talking to patients in a non-judgemental and accessible manner about sexual issues. • Learn about the assessment and management of risk. • Become familiar with the diagnosis and management of common STIs. • Gain experience in contraceptive counselling and handling unwanted pregnancies. • Learn about psychosexual problems and the treatments and sources of support available. • Understand what steps can be taken to make services more accessible to younger people – find out about their concerns in accessing services. • Find out about the management of HIV and Hepatitis B/C. • Learn how to recognise and treat genital warts. • Become practised at vaginal and rectal examinations and taking cervical samples and swabs
Medical specialties (e.g. cardiovascular, chest medicine, diabetes, endocrinology, renal, oncology, etc.)	Read the clinical example statements of relevance to the particular placement, such as: 3.12 *Cardiovascular Health* 3.13 *Digestive Health* 3.17 *Care of People with Metabolic Problems* 3.18 *Care of People with Neurological Problems* 3.19 *Respiratory Health*	• Medical specialty placements are good opportunities for learning in depth about the specialist management of the common conditions that are mostly managed in primary care (e.g. Type 2 diabetes, asthma, COPD, hypothyroidism). • These placements are also good for learning about the important but less common medical conditions (e.g. cancer), as you will encounter patients with these conditions more frequently over a shorter period of time than in general practice

Placement	Make sure you read	Hints and tips for learning the curriculum
Medical specialties (e.g. cardiovascular, chest medicine, diabetes, endocrinology, renal, oncology, etc.)	Read the clinical example statements of relevance to the particular placement, such as: 3.12 *Cardiovascular Health* 3.13 *Digestive Health* 3.17 *Care of People with Metabolic Problems* 3.18 *Care of People with Neurological Problems* 3.19 *Respiratory Health*	• Try to spend time with different members of the multidisciplinary team (e.g. the specialist nurses) – they often act as a bridge between the patient and the hospital, and will provide an insight that will prove useful when you are in general practice. • Gain experience in interpreting diagnostic tests that are also performed in primary care (e.g. ECGs, events monitors, lung function tests) as well as gaining an awareness of the role of more specialised tests. • Practise your clinical examination skills and develop routines that can be adapted to a ten-minute GP consultation
Obstetrics and gynaecology	3.06 *Women's Health* *Also read 3.02* Genetics in Primary Care *for information on prenatal testing*	• Outpatients offer a great opportunity to learn about the investigation and management of many common gynaecological conditions – e.g. menstrual problems, post-menopausal bleeding, PCOS, pelvic pain, infertility (see statement). • Learn about the management of early pregnancy problems such as pain and bleeding (including suspected ectopic pregnancy) and hyperemesis – you will see these commonly in general practice. • Prenatal diagnosis – try to spend some time in the PND unit and understand the choices available to parents and how these are best communicated. • Routine antenatal care – you must become well practised in performing a routine antenatal check and understand how to monitor and manage common pregnancy complications

Continued over

Placement	Make sure you read	Hints and tips for learning the curriculum
Obstetrics and gynaecology *(continued)*	3.06 *Women's Health* *Also read 3.02* Genetics in Primary Care *for information on prenatal testing*	• On the labour ward, make sure you witness the range of different deliveries – and learn how to do a vaginal delivery, just in case! • There are many opportunities to improve vaginal, speculum and pelvic examination skills. • Learn how to fit a ring pessary
Ophthalmology	3.16 *Care of People with Eye Problems*	• Become familiar with diagnosing and managing common eye emergencies – spend time in eye casualty as patients frequently present in general practice with similar conditions. • Learn about the management of common long-term eye conditions, such as glaucoma and macular degeneration. • Find out about the services and support available for people with visual impairment. • Remember you are very unlikely to have access to a slit lamp in general practice – learn how to examine patients with an ophthalmoscope!
Paediatrics	3.04 *Care of Children and Young People*	• This placement provides valuable experience in assessing sick children in a supervised environment, so you can learn safely to distinguish the snotty-but-well child from the seriously ill child. • Gain an understanding of how children and adults differ in their illness behaviour and how apparently sick children can rapidly improve – and how apparently well children can rapidly deteriorate. Learn how to elicit parental concerns and incorporate these into your decisions. • Learn how to manage consultations with parents and how to adapt your consultation skills to suit children of different ages

Placement	Make sure you read	Hints and tips for learning the curriculum
Paediatrics (continued)	3.04 *Care of Children and Young People*	• Find out about the management of common long-term conditions affecting children and how to best support parents with chronically ill or disabled children. • Observe normal (and abnormal) child behaviour and development. • Spend time with community paediatricians and child health nurses. • Learn about the issues around transition and how these can be managed – from childhood to adolescence to adulthood. • Practise performing routine 'baby checks' and get experienced paediatricians to teach you their techniques for examining infants and young children
Psychiatry	3.10 *Care of People with Mental Health Problems* 3.14 *Care of People Who Misuse Drugs and Alcohol*	• This placement provides valuable opportunities to learn about the assessment and management of more severe cases of common mental health problems. • On-call provides useful opportunities to learn about the assessment and management of mental health emergencies and how to deal with the patient in crisis. • Learn how to support patients in recovery, promote mental health resilience and monitor for signs of relapse. • Become familiar with the commonly used treatments, including the range of psychological therapies and support services available. • Spend time with community psychiatric nurses, psychologists and mental health social workers

Continued over

Placement	Make sure you read	Hints and tips for learning the curriculum
Psychiatry *(continued)*	3.10 *Care of People with Mental Health Problems* 3.14 *Care of People Who Misuse Drugs and Alcohol*	• Try to spend time with the community addictions service. • Learn about the Mental Health Act and the GP's role in this. • Become familiar with assessing the risk of suicide and self-harm, and responding effectively and appropriately to those at risk of harm
Research or academic post	2.4 *Enhancing Professional Knowledge*	• Develop your skills in evidence-based medicine including interpretation of original data. • Undertake an audit or quality improvement project. • Focus on developing your leadership and educational skills
Rheumatology and/or MSK medicine	3.20 *Care of People with Musculoskeletal Problems*	• This is a great opportunity to learn how to recognise the patterns of symptoms that suggest inflammatory or non-inflammatory disease. • Become familiar with the common diagnostic tests in rheumatological conditions and how to interpret these. • Learn techniques for prioritising problems in patients who present with lots of aches and pains. • Learn the indications for and monitoring of disease-modifying drugs and other treatment options for patients with rheumatological conditions. • Spend time with specialist nurses and find out how to better support patients with long-term pain and disability

Placement	Make sure you read	Hints and tips for learning the curriculum
Rheumatology and/or MSK medicine *(continued)*	3.20 *Care of People with Musculoskeletal Problems*	• Practise musculoskeletal examinations and develop a routine for examining a patient that can be adapted for a ten-minute GP consultation. • Learn how to carry out commonly performed joint injections (e.g. shoulders and knees)

Appendix 2
MRCGP Consultation Observation Tool (COT)

COT performance criteria	Insufficient evidence _I_	Needs further development _N_	Competent _C_	Excellent _E_
1 Encourages the patient's contribution				
2 Responds to cues				
3 Places complaint in appropriate psychosocial contexts				
4 Explores patient's health understanding				
5 Includes or excludes likely relevant significant condition				
6 Appropriate physical or mental state examination				
7 Makes an appropriate working diagnosis				
8 Explains the problem in appropriate language				
9 Seeks to confirm patient's understanding				
10 Appropriate management plan				
11 Patient is given the opportunity to be involved in significant management decisions				
12 Makes effective use of resources				
13 Conditions and interval for follow-up are specified				
Overall assessment:	_I_	_N_	_C_	_E_

Feedback and recommendations for further development:

Note: a detailed guide to the performance criteria is available on the RCGP website (www.rcgp.org.uk).

Appendix 3
Common GP topics mapped to the relevant curriculum statements

The following table lists topics commonly learned or taught in educational and training activities related to general practice. These have been mapped to their relevant RCGP curriculum contextual and clinical examples statements,[i] which have been summarised in Chapter 6, 'The applied knowledge'.

Statement 1.0 *Being a General Practitioner* is the core curriculum statement and can be used as a wide-ranging resource for most educational activities in general practice. As it is so wide-ranging, it is not included here. The key competencies and expertise required of a GP are covered in depth in Chapter 5, 'The core curriculum'.

Clinical topics where the relevant curriculum statement is very obvious have not been included (e.g. skin rashes are covered by statement 3.21: *Care of People with Skin Problems*).

Common GP topics	*Relevant contextual and clinical example statements*
Abdominal pain (chronic)	3.13 *Digestive Health*
	3.04 *Care of Children and Young People*
Accounts and book-keeping	2.03 *The GP in the Wider Professional Environment*
Acute abdomen	3.03 *Care of Acutely Ill People*
	3.13 *Digestive Health*
Adult learning skills	2.04 *Enhancing Professional Knowledge*
Alcohol problems	3.14 *Care of People Who Misuse Drugs and Alcohol*
Anaemia	3.X *The Rest of General Practice**
Antenatal care	3.06 *Women's Health*
Antenatal testing	3.02 *Genetics in Primary Care*
	3.06 *Women's Health*
Anxiety and panic attacks	3.10 *Care of People with Mental Health Problems*

i Royal College of General Practitioners revised curriculum statements. Available at: www.rcgp.org.uk/curriculum [accessed May 2012].

Appointment systems	2.03 *The GP in the Wider Professional Environment*
Arthritis	3.20 *Care of People with Musculoskeletal Problems*
Asthma	3.03 *Care of Acutely Ill People*
	3.04 *Care of Children and Young People*
	3.19 *Respiratory Health*
Audit	2.02 *Patient Safety and Quality of Care*
Backache	3.20 *Care of People with Musculoskeletal Problems*
Behavioural problems	3.04 *Care of Children and Young People*
Beliefs and attitudes	2.01 *The GP Consultation in Practice*
Blood pressure monitoring	3.12 *Cardiovascular Health*
Bowel cancer	3.09 *End-of-Life Care*
	3.13 *Digestive Health*
Breaking bad news	2.01 *The GP Consultation in Practice*
Breast disorders	3.06 *Women's Health*
Breastfeeding	3.04 *Care of Children and Young People*
Breathlessness	3.03 *Care of Acutely Ill People*
	3.12 *Cardiovascular Health*
	3.19 *Respiratory Health*
Cancer investigation and referral	2.01 *The GP Consultation in Practice*
	3.09 *End-of-Life Care*
Cancer screening programmes	3.01 *Healthy People: promoting health and preventing disease*
	3.09 *End-of-Life Care*
Carers (role and support of)	3.09 *End-of-Life Care*
	3.11 *Care of People with Intellectual Disability*
Cervical smears	3.01 *Healthy People: promoting health and preventing disease*
	3.09 *End-of-Life Care*
	3.06 *Women's Health*

Change in bowel habit	3.09 *End-of-Life Care*
	3.13 *Digestive Health*
Chaperones	3.06 *Women's Health*
	3.07 *Men's Health*
Chest pain	3.03 *Care of Acutely Ill People*
	3.12 *Cardiovascular Health*
Child development	3.01 *Healthy People: promoting health and preventing disease*
	3.04 *Care of Children and Young People*
Child protection	2.02 *Patient Safety and Quality of Care*
	3.04 *Care of Children and Young People*
Chronic disease management	3.05 *Care of Older Adults*
	3.17 *Care of People with Metabolic Problems*
Common illnesses in childhood	3.04 *Care of Children and Young People*
	3.15 *Care of People with ENT, Oral and Facial Problems*
Communication skills	2.01 *The GP Consultation in Practice*
Community midwife	3.06 *Women's Health*
Community/district nurses and local health services	3.01 *Healthy People: promoting health and preventing disease*
	3.05 *Care of Older Adults*
	3.09 *End-of-Life Care*
	3.10 *Care of People with Mental Health Problems*
	3.11 *Care of People with Intellectual Disability*
	3.20 *Care of People with Musculoskeletal Problems*
Co-morbidity	3.05 *Care of Older Adults*
Computers in general practice	2.02 *Patient Safety and Quality of Care*
Confidentiality	2.02 *Patient Safety and Quality of Care*
Conflicts of interest and probity	2.01 *The GP Consultation in Practice*
	2.02 *Patient Safety and Quality of Care*

Consent	3.10 *Care of People with Mental Health Problems*
	3.11 *Care of People with Intellectual Disability*
	3.21 *Care of People with Skin Problems*
Consultation models	2.01 *The GP Consultation in Practice*
Contraception	3.06 *Women's Health*
	3.08 *Sexual Health*
Contracts – GMS and PMS	2.03 *The GP in the Wider Professional Environment*
Controlled drugs	2.02 *Patient Safety and Quality of Care*
COPD	3.19 *Respiratory Health*
Coroner	3.09 *End-of-Life Care*
Critical appraisal and EBM	2.04 *Enhancing Professional Knowledge*
Cultural aspects of general practice	2.01 *The GP Consultation in Practice*
Cystitis	3.06 *Women's Health*
Data protection	2.02 *Patient Safety and Quality of Care*
Deafness	3.15 *Care of People with ENT, Oral and Facial Problems*
Dealing with uncertainty	2.01 *The GP Consultation in Practice*
Death certification and cremation	3.09 *End-of-Life Care*
Decision-making skills	2.01 *The GP Consultation in Practice*
Delegation	2.03 *The GP in the Wider Professional Environment*
Depression	3.10 *Care of People with Mental Health Problems*
Diabetes	3.17 *Care of People with Metabolic Problems*
Diarrhoea and vomiting	3.03 *Care of Acutely Ill People*
	3.04 *Care of Children and Young People*
	3.13 *Digestive Health*
Difficult patients	2.01 *The GP Consultation in Practice*
Difficulties with colleagues	2.02 *Patient Safety and Quality of Care*
Dispensing drugs	2.02 *Patient Safety and Quality of Care*

Down's syndrome	3.02 *Genetics in Primary Care*
Drug abuse	3.14 *Care of People Who Misuse Drugs and Alcohol*
Drug companies and reps	2.01 *The GP Consultation in Practice*
	2.02 *Patient Safety and Quality of Care*
Dyspepsia and reflux	3.13 *Digestive Health*
ECG use and interpretation	3.12 *Cardiovascular Health*
Eliciting skills	2.01 *The GP Consultation in Practice*
Emergency equipment and drugs	3.03 *Care of Acutely Ill People*
Emergency procedures and skills	3.03 *Care of Acutely Ill People*
Employment law	2.03 *The GP in the Wider Professional Environment*
Enuresis	3.04 *Care of Children and Young People*
Epidemiology	3.01 *Healthy People: promoting health and preventing disease*
Epilepsy	3.18 *Care of People with Neurological Problems*
	3.04 *Care of Children and Young People*
Ethical committees	2.04 *Enhancing Professional Knowledge*
Ethnicity	2.01 *The GP Consultation in Practice*
Euthanasia	2.01 *The GP Consultation in Practice*
	2.02 *Patient Safety and Quality of Care*
Family planning	3.08 *Sexual Health*
Feedback, giving and receiving	2.04 *Enhancing Professional Knowledge*
Fits and faints	3.18 *Care of People with Neurological Problems*
Glandular fever	3.04 *Care of Children and Young People*
GMC and *Good Medical Practice*	2.02 *Patient Safety and Quality of Care*
GUM and STIs	3.08 *Sexual Health*
Gynaecological problems	3.06 *Women's Health*

Haematology	3.X *The Rest of General Practice**
	3.09 *End-of-Life Care*
Haematuria	3.06 *Women's Health*
	3.07 *Men's Health*
Headaches	3.18 *Care of People with Neurological Problems*
Health and safety	2.02 *Patient Safety and Quality of Care*
	2.03 *The GP in the Wider Professional Environment*
Health promotion	3.01 *Healthy People: promoting health and preventing disease*
Health visitors	3.04 *Care of Children and Young People*
Heart failure	3.12 *Cardiovascular Health*
Hernias and abdominal masses	3.13 *Digestive Health*
Hidden presentation of illness	2.01 *The GP Consultation in Practice*
HIV and AIDS	3.08 *Sexual Health*
Home visits	2.01 *The GP Consultation in Practice*
Hypertension	3.12 *Cardiovascular Health*
Immunisation and vaccination	3.01 *Healthy People: promoting health and preventing disease*
	3.04 *Care of Children and Young People*
Inequalities in health care	2.01 *The GP Consultation in Practice*
	3.01 *Healthy People: promoting health and preventing disease*
Infectious diseases	3.X *The Rest of General Practice**
Infertility – female	3.06 *Women's Health*
Infertility – male	3.07 *Men's Health*
Influenza campaigns	3.01 *Healthy People: promoting health and preventing disease*
Investigations in primary care	2.04 *Enhancing Professional Knowledge*
Lung cancer	3.09 *End-of-Life Care*
	3.19 *Respiratory Health*

Management of change	2.02 *Patient Safety and Quality of Care*
	2.04 *Enhancing Professional Knowledge*
	2.03 *The GP in the Wider Professional Environment*
Management theory and practice	2.03 *The GP in the Wider Professional Environment*
Maternity leave	3.06 *Women's Health*
Medically unexplained symptoms	3.10 *Care of People with Mental Health Problems*
	3.X *The Rest of General Practice**
Meetings	2.02 *Patient Safety and Quality of Care*
	2.03 *The GP in the Wider Professional Environment*
Meningitis	3.03 *Care of Acutely Ill People*
	3.04 *Care of Children and Young People*
	3.18 *Care of People with Neurological Problems*
Menstrual problems	3.06 *Women's Health*
Mental Health Act	3.10 *Care of People with Mental Health Problems*
Migraine	3.18 *Care of People with Neurological Problems*
Minor illnesses in adults	3.13 *Digestive Health*
	3.15 *Care of People with ENT, Oral and Facial Problems*
	3.19 *Respiratory Health*
	3.21 *Care of People with Skin Problems*
Minor injuries	3.20 *Care of People with Musculoskeletal Problems*
	3.21 *Care of People with Skin Problems*
Minor surgery	3.21 *Care of People with Skin Problems*
Moles	3.21 *Care of People with Skin Problems*
Motivation	2.03 *The GP in the Wider Professional Environment*
Multiple sclerosis	3.18 *Care of People with Neurological Problems*
Neck lumps	3.15 *Care of People with ENT, Oral and Facial Problems*

Obesity	3.01 *Healthy People: promoting health and preventing disease*
	3.17 *Care of People with Metabolic Problems*
Obstetrics	3.06 *Women's Health*
Occupational health	3.X *The Rest of General Practice**
Off legs	3.X *The Rest of General Practice**
Oral contraception	3.06 *Women's Health*
	3.08 *Sexual Health*
Osteoporosis	3.06 *Women's Health*
	3.17 *Care of People with Metabolic Problems*
Palliative care	3.09 *End-of-Life Care*
Parkinson's disease	3.18 *Care of People with Neurological Problems*
Partnership agreements	2.03 *The GP in the Wider Professional Environment*
Partnership organisation	2.03 *The GP in the Wider Professional Environment*
Patient information leaflets	2.01 *The GP Consultation in Practice*
Patient participation	2.02 *Patient Safety and Quality of Care*
Pensions and superannuation	2.03 *The GP in the Wider Professional Environment*
Peripheral vascular disease	3.12 *Cardiovascular Health*
Physiotherapy	3.20 *Care of People with Musculoskeletal Problems*
Postnatal care	3.06 *Women's Health*
Practice finances	2.03 *The GP in the Wider Professional Environment*
Practice managers	2.02 *Patient Safety and Quality of Care*
	2.03 *The GP in the Wider Professional Environment*
Practice nurses	3.01 *Healthy People: promoting health and preventing disease*
	3.12 *Cardiovascular Health*
	3.17 *Care of People with Metabolic Problems*
	3.19 *Respiratory Health*
Premises	2.03 *The GP in the Wider Professional Environment*

Prescribing monitoring	2.02 *Patient Safety and Quality of Care*
Prevention	3.01 *Healthy People: promoting health and preventing disease*
Problem solving	2.01 *The GP Consultation in Practice*
Prostate disorders	3.07 *Men's Health*
Protocols and guidelines	2.04 *Enhancing Professional Knowledge*
Psychiatric emergencies	3.03 *Care of Acutely Ill People*
	3.10 *Care of People with Mental Health Problems*
Psychosexual problems	3.06 *Women's Health*
	3.07 *Men's Health*
	3.08 *Sexual Health*
Quality assurance	2.02 *Patient Safety and Quality of Care*
	2.03 *The GP in the Wider Professional Environment*
Record keeping	2.02 *Patient Safety and Quality of Care*
Red eye	3.16 *Care of People with Eye Problems*
Referral systems	2.01 *The GP Consultation in Practice*
	3.09 *End-of-Life Care*
Relationship difficulties	3.10 *Care of People with Mental Health Problems*
Relationships with colleagues	2.02 *Patient Safety and Quality of Care*
Relationships with patients	2.01 *The GP Consultation in Practice*
Renal problems	3.06 *Women's Health*
	3.07 *Men's Health*
	3.X *The Rest of General Practice**
Repeat prescriptions	2.02 *Patient Safety and Quality of Care*
Research	2.04 *Enhancing Professional Knowledge*
Residential and nursing care	3.05 *Care of Older Adults*
Respect for patients' dignity	2.01 *The GP Consultation in Practice*
Resuscitation and BLS	3.03 *Care of Acutely Ill People*

Screening programmes	3.01 *Healthy People: promoting health and preventing disease*
Services for the disabled	3.05 *Care of Older Adults*
	3.10 *Care of People with Mental Health Problems*
Sickness certification	2.01 *The GP Consultation in Practice*
Significant Event Analysis	2.02 *Patient Safety and Quality of Care*
Smoking	3.01 *Healthy People: promoting health and preventing disease*
Sports injuries	3.20 *Care of People with Musculoskeletal Problems*
Statistics	2.04 *Enhancing Professional Knowledge*
Sterilisation	3.06 *Women's Health*
	3.07 *Men's Health*
	3.08 *Sexual Health*
Stroke	3.05 *Care of Older Adults*
	3.12 *Cardiovascular Health*
	3.18 *Care of People with Neurological Problems*
Suicide and deliberate self-harm	3.10 *Care of People with Mental Health Problems*
Surgery	3.X *The Rest of General Practice**
Teaching skills	2.04 *Enhancing Professional Knowledge*
Teenage health care	3.04 *Care of Children and Young People*
	3.08 *Sexual Health*
	3.14 *Care of People Who Misuse Drugs and Alcohol*
Telephone consultations	2.01 *The GP Consultation in Practice*
	2.02 *Patient Safety and Quality of Care*
Terminal care	3.09 *End-of-Life Care*
Termination of pregnancy	3.06 *Women's Health*
	3.08 *Sexual Health*
Thyroid disease	3.17 *Care of People with Metabolic Problems*
Time management	2.01 *The GP Consultation in Practice*

Travel advice and vaccinations	3.X *The Rest of General Practice**
Uncertainty, dealing with	2.01 *The GP Consultation in Practice*
Urinary disorders	3.06 *Women's Health*
	3.07 *Men's Health*
Use of time as a diagnostic tool	2.01 *The GP Consultation in Practice*
Venous thrombosis	3.12 *Cardiovascular Health*
Vertigo and dizziness	3.15 *Care of People with ENT, Oral and Facial Problems*
	3.18 *Care of People with Neurological Problems*
Violence	2.02 *Patient Safety and Quality of Care*
	3.06 *Women's Health*
	3.07 *Men's Health*
	3.10 *Care of People with Mental Health Problems*
Visual impairment and blindness	3.16 *Care of People with Eye Problems*
Warfarin monitoring	3.X *The Rest of General Practice**
Work–life balance	2.02 *Patient Safety and Quality of Care*
X-rays and imaging services	2.04 *Enhancing Professional Knowledge*

*3.X: *The Rest of General Practice* is not an official curriculum statement. It was created in *The Condensed Curriculum Guide* to contain primary care topics that are not explicitly described in an existing curriculum statement.

Index

A&E placements 306
abdominal pain 317
abortion *see* termination of pregnancy
academic posts 3, 312
access to care
  children and young people 191
  drugs and alcohol misusers 252
  men 211
  older people 197
  people with hearing impairment 260
  people with intellectual disability 238
  psychological therapies 231
  sexual health services 218, 220
  women 205
accident prevention 190
accounts 317
acronyms 42
acute general medical placements 304
acute illness 178
  condensed know-how 182–4
  condensed knowledge 178–80
  condensed resources 185
  condensed skills 180–2
  dangerous diagnoses 186
addictions *see* alcohol misuse; drug misuse
Adding Years to Life 198
adolescence 191
adult learning skills 158, 161, 317
adverse events 146–7
advocacy for patients 90
Age UK 199
ageing 196
agendas
  conflicting 138
  non-medical 114
AIDS (acquired immunodeficiency syndrome) 215, 217, 322
AKT *see* Applied Knowledge Test
alarm symptoms *see* red flags
alcohol misuse 250
  brief intervention model 255
  condensed know-how 252–3

condensed knowledge 250–1
condensed resources 254–5
condensed skills 252
algorithm completion questions 44
anaemia 317
anaphylaxis kits 104
anger, feelings of 20
annual health checks, people with intellectual disability 238, 239
Annual Review of Competence Progression 70, 72–3
antenatal care 317
  genetic screening 176
antibiotic prescribing, ENT conditions 259
antiretroviral therapy 217
anxiety 317
application features 11
applied knowledge 75
Applied Knowledge Test (AKT) 38
  content guide 46
  preparation 45–6
  question sources 45
  question types 43–4
appointment systems 318
appraisal 34
apprenticeship 7–8
areas of competence 15, 38, 39–40, 77–9
  community orientation 111–16
  comprehensive approach 106
  holistic approach 117–18
  learning and teaching tips 79
  person-centred approach 92–7
  primary care management 80–91
  problem-solving skills 98–105
  use in planning learning 127
arthritis *see* musculoskeletal conditions
Arthritis Research UK 291
aspirin, in patients with diabetes 270
asthma
  self-management 280, 281
  see also respiratory health
attitudes 48, 318
  assessment 40
attitudinal features 119, 122–4

attorney, power of 198
audit 114, 144, 318
audit cycle 150
automated external defibrillation
  (AED) training 67
autonomy 94, 142
    in acute illness 183, 184
autosomal dominant disorders 173
awareness-raising 242

backache 318
Bandolier
    evidence-based medicine website
    167
    men's health collection 213
    research terms glossary 162
basic life support 104, 325
behavioural change 169
behavioural problems 318
behaviours
    assessment 40
    Clinical Skills Assessment 50–2
beliefs 318
beneficence 142
bereavement 225, 226
BetterTesting 135
biopsychosocial whole 117
blindness 262, 265–6, 327
blood pressure monitoring 318
BMJ Learning 135
book-keeping 317
borderline group method 47
bowel cancer 318
breaking bad news 318
breast disorders 318
breastfeeding 318
breathlessness 318
brief intervention model, alcohol
  misuse 255
British Association for Sexual Health
  and HIV 221
British Association of
  Dermatologists 296
British Geriatrics Society 199
British Institute of Learning
  Disabilities (BILD) 239
British Society for Human Genetics
  177
British Society for Sexual Medicine
  221
British Thoracic Society guidelines
  282

burnout 124

cancer investigation and referral 318
cancer resources 227
cancer screening 318
    colorectal cancer 248
    see also screening
cannabis use 250
    see also drug misuse
capacity 139, 239
cardio-pulmonary resuscitation
  (CPR) training 67
cardiovascular health 240
    condensed know-how 242–3
    condensed knowledge 240–1
    condensed resources 243–4
    condensed skills 242
cardiovascular risk prediction charts
  244
care pathways 88
Care Programme Approach (CPA)
  232
carers 318
case analysis 24–5
    problem-based 26
case-based discussion (CbD) 57, 58,
  61–3
case-finding strategies, women's
  health 205
cervical smears 318
change in bowel habit 319
change management 144, 323
Changing Faces 296
chaperones 206, 319
chest pain 319
child development 319
child protection 319
child safeguarding 191–2
children, care of 187
    condensed know-how 190–3
    condensed knowledge 187–9
    condensed resources 193–4
    condensed skills 189
    contraception and sexual health
    220
    mental health 232
    musculoskeletal conditions 286
    paediatric placements 310–11
    visual impairment 265
'Choose and Book' system 88
chromosome anomalies 172, 177
chronic disease management 81–2, 319

nurse-led clinics 242
chronic obstructive airways disease
(COPD) 320
    see also respiratory health
clinical coding systems 138
clinical example statements 11, 12,
13–14
clinical governance 143
Clinical Governance Support Teams
149
clinical management 39
    care of older people 195
Clinical Skills Assessment (CSA) 38,
46–7, 51
    areas covered 48
    difference between passing and
    failing 50–2
    examples of cases 48
    marking 47
    preparation 47, 49–50
clinical skills demonstration 48
clinical skills development 84
clinical supervisors 41–2
Clinical Supervisor's Report (CSR)
56, 58, 68–9
codes of practice 148
coding systems 138
College of Sexual and Relationship
Therapists (COSRT) 222
commissioning cycle 166
commissioning of services 89,
113–14, 115–16, 154
    RCGP online course 170
communication skills 39, 86, 89, 94,
143, 167, 319
    acute illness 180
    care of children and young
    people 189
    care of older people 195
    Clinical Skills Assessment 51
    cultural differences 50
    end-of-life care 224
    ENT problems 258
    genetic conditions 174
    language problems 50
    men's health 210
    people with intellectual disability
    238
    within the practice 152
community delivery of health care
154
community influences 120, 153

community knowledge 99
community midwife 319
community nurses 319
community orientation 39, 79, 111–16
community pharmacists, learning
opportunities 28
co-morbidity 106, 196, 319
    in diabetes 270
competencies 11, 14–15
    see also areas of competence
competency, evidence of 53
complaints system 148
complex skills 26, 39
complexity of health problems 109
comprehensive approach 48, 79, 106
    health promotion and disease
    prevention 107–9
    managing multiple pathologies
    106–7
    variety of approaches to patients
    109–10
compromise 91
compulsory admission and
treatment 184
computer use 319
concordance 232
    cardiovascular medication 242
condensed statements 131
confidence rating 24
confidence rating scale 132
confidentiality 139, 319
    children and young people 192,
    193
    genetic conditions 177
    older people 198
    sexual health 219, 220
    women's issues 206
conflicts 138, 319
connecting, consultation skills 93
consent 94, 139, 320
    capacity for 239
consultant ward rounds, learning
opportunities 29
consultation analysis 18–19, 49, 64
consultation models 140, 320
consultation observation tool (COT)
18, 57, 58, 63–4, 315
consultation skills 39, 81, 89, 136–8,
158
    acute illness 181
    children and young people 189
    condensed know-how 138–9

condensed resources 141
digestive health 247
drug and alcohol misuse 252
ENT problems 258
ethical principles 142
genetic conditions 174
health promotion 167
intellectual disability 237
mental health problems 230
metabolic problems 269
musculoskeletal conditions 288
neurological problems 276
older people 195
person-centred approach 93–4
respiratory health 280
sexual health 217
skin problems 294–5
consultation times 120
contextual features 119–21
contextual statements 12, 13
continuing professional development
  (CPD) 6, 33–4, 40, 126
continuity of care 96, 139
    in acute illness 183
    in mental health 232
contraception 216, 217, 219, 220, 320
    resources 221, 222
contracts 153, 320
controlled drugs 320
coordination of care, people with
  intellectual disability 237
core competences 5
core curriculum 75
core of general practice 77
core statement 12
coronary heart disease
    NSF 244
    see also cardiovascular health
coroners 320
'corridor consultations' 124
cost–benefit analysis 105
cost-efficiency 105
counselling skills
    end-of-life care 224
    sexual health 217
    smoking cessation 280
counselling teaching method 163
counter-transference 123
courses 34
cremation 320
Criminal Records Bureau disclosure
  191

critical appraisal 125, 157, 320
critical appraisal workbooks 46
critical events analysis 25
Cruse Bereavement Care 226
CSA see Clinical Skills Assessment
CSR see Clinical Supervisor's Report
cultural beliefs, genetic conditions
  176
cultural issues 50, 118, 320
    in emergency situations 184
    ENT problems 260
    in mental health 233
    older people 198
    sexual health 220
    women's health 206
curriculum
    2012 revision 5
    everyday use 9
    hidden 9
    informal 8
    initial development 4
    relationship to MRCGP
    assessments 40, 41
    review process 4–5
    role in GP training 5–6
    use in training difficulties 30, 31
    what it is 3
    for whom it is designed 3
curriculum framework 11
curriculum resources 134
curriculum statements 11, 13–14, 15
    clinical examples 12
    contextual statements 11, 12
    core statement 12
    internet access 13
    as a teaching resource 29–30
cystitis 320

dangerous diagnoses 186
data gathering and interpretation 39
    Clinical Skills Assessment 51
data protection 320
deafness 260, 320
death certification 183, 198, 320
decision making 39, 320
    in acute illness 181
decision-making capacity 139
decision-making tools 99
defibrillators 104
delegation 320
dementia, resources 199
depression 320

in chronic diseases 271
NICE quality standard 233
dermatology 292
    condensed know-how 295–6
    condensed knowledge 292–4
    condensed resources 296
    condensed skills 294–5
dermatology placements 304–5
diabetes mellitus 267, 320
    condensed know-how 270–1
    condensed knowledge 267–9
    condensed resources 271–2
    condensed skills 269
diabetic retinopathy screening 265
diagnoses, dangerous 186
diagnostic overshadowing 235, 238
diagnostic skills, acute illness 182
diarrhoea 320
didactic teaching method 163
difficult patients 320
difficulties with colleagues 320
digestive health 245
    condensed know-how 248
    condensed knowledge 245–7
    condensed resources 249
    condensed skills 247–8
dignity, respect for 325
Diploma of the Faculty of Family
    Planning and Reproductive Care
    221
direct observation of procedural
    skills (DOPS) 57, 59–60
Directgov, information for disabled
    people 239
disabilities, children and young
    people 193
disability services 326
Disabled Living Foundation 291
disabled parking badges 289
disease prevention see preventive
    activities
disease registers 97
dispensing drugs 320
district nurses 319
    learning opportunities 28
dizziness 327
'DNAs', children and young people
    191
'Do Not Resuscitate' orders 183
doctor–patient relationship
    autonomy 94
    boundaries 95

communication of findings 94
consultation skills 93–4
continuity of care 96
gender issues 206, 212
subjectivity 95
doctor's bag 180
Doctors.net 46, 135, 185
domestic violence 205
    resources 207
DOPS see direct observation of
    procedural skills
Down's syndrome 321
driving
    disabled parking badges 289
    DVLA guidelines 199, 243, 266,
    276
    older people 198
drug-associated skin problems 295
drug companies and reps 321
drug misuse 250, 321
    condensed know-how 252–3
    condensed knowledge 250–1
    condensed resources 254–5
    condensed skills 252
DS1500 225
dyspepsia 321

ear, nose and throat (ENT)
    problems
    condensed know-how 259–61
    condensed knowledge 256–8
    condensed resources 261
    condensed skills 258–9
ear, nose and throat placements 307
early general practice placements
    304
eating disorders 193
ECGs 321
educational meetings, learning
    opportunities 29
educational supervisors 41
    reports 72
educators, value of the curriculum 3
e-GP 134, 170
    on care of children 194
    on care of older people 199
    on emergency care 185
    on end-of-life care 226
    on eye problems 266
    genetics resources 177
    on intellectual disabilities 239
    on metabolic problems 271

on musculoskeletal conditions 290

on sexual health 221

on women's health 207

elderly care placements 305

elderly people *see* older adults, care of

e-learning modules 46, 49

on end-of-life care 226

eliciting skills 321

embarrassing problems website 213

emergencies

urgent intervention 103–4

see also acute illness

emergency equipment 180, 183, 321

emergency medicine placements 306

emergency procedures and skills 321

emergency protocols 182

employment law 321

employment policies 154

EMQ *see* extended matching questions

endocrine problems *see* metabolic problems

end-of-life care 223

condensed know-how 225–6

condensed knowledge 223–4

condensed resources 226–7

condensed skills 224–5

end-of-life care placements 307

Enhancing Professional Knowledge 156

condensed know-how 159–62

condensed knowledge 156–7

condensed resources 162–3

condensed skills 158–9

enuresis 321

environmental impact of services 155

epidemiological knowledge 98–9, 111

epidemiology 80–1, 321

epilepsy 321

driving 276

medication issues 276

see also neurological problems

episodic continuity 96

ePortfolio 52–3, 53

cardio-pulmonary resuscitation training 67

case-based discussion 61–3

consultation observation tool 63–4

direct observation of procedural

skills 59–60

evidence collection 53–4

naturally occurring evidence 54–5

writing learning log entries 55, 56

mini-clinical evaluation exercise 61

multi-source feedback 66–7

out-of-hours experience 67–8

patient satisfaction questionnaires 65

templates 54

Workplace-Based Assessment tools 55–9, 58

Equality Act 2010 260

equality issues 154

errors 146

essential application features 15, 119

attitudinal 122–4

contextual 119–21

scientific 125–6

ethical committees 321

ethical practice 40, 48, 122, 136, 139

drug and alcohol misuse 253

end-of-life care 226

four key principles 142

genetic conditions 177

healthcare provision 169

management and leadership issues 155

mental health 233

neurological problems 277

older people 198

sexual health 220

ethical tensions 109, 148

ethics, personal 124

ethnicity 321

impact on health 112

euthanasia 321

evidence-based practice 84, 107, 139, 156, 158, 164

influencing factors 159–60

evidence collection 53–4

naturally occurring evidence 54–5

timetable 71

writing learning log entries 55

exceptional potential consultation model 140

experiential learning 17, 18–19

expert patients 139, 290

explaining diagnoses and treatments 49

extended matching questions (EMQ) 43

eye problems 262
   condensed know-how 265–6
   condensed knowledge 262–4
   condensed resources 266
   condensed skills 264
   ophthalmology placements 310

Faculty of Public Health of the Royal College of Physicians 113

faints 321

familial hypercholesterolaemia 176

family history 100, 172, 175

family planning 321

feedback 30, 32, 49, 321
   to colleagues 158
   multi-source feedback 66–7
   patient satisfaction questionnaires 65
   principles of constructive feedback 32

financial aspects of practice 153

financial frameworks 120

financial support, people with intellectual disability 238, 239

First Practice Management 155

fit notes 291

fitness to practise 40

fits 321

five-checkpoint consultation model 140

folk model of illness 93
   skill development 138

formative assessment 30, 32

FPA 221

FRAMES brief intervention model 255

free-text questions 44

frequent attenders, mental health 232

GAD-7 assessment 234

gastroenterology see digestive health

'gatekeeper' role 91, 115

General Medical Council (GMC)
   Good Medical Practice 77, 321
   guidance on end-of-life care 226
   guidance on learning disabilities 239

generic competencies 77

genetic testing 175

genetics 172
   condensed know-how 175–7
   condensed knowledge 172–4
   condensed resources 177
   condensed skills 174–5

genetics services 175

genito-urinary medicine 321

genito-urinary medicine placements 308

glandular fever 321

glaucoma screening 265

GMC see General Medical Council

Good Medical Practice, GMC 77, 321

Good Medical Practice for General Practitioners, RCGP 77

gout 267
   condensed know-how 270–1
   condensed knowledge 267–9

GP press 33

GP trainers, role 7–8

GP training
   organisation 6–7
   role of the curriculum 5–6

GPnotebook 46, 135, 185

GP in the Wider Professional Environment
   condensed know-how 153–5
   condensed resources 155
   condensed skills 151–2

Great Ormond Street website 194

group learning 27

growth and development 191

guardians of statements 5

guidelines 325
   see also National Institute for Health and Clinical Excellence (NICE); National Service Frameworks; SIGN guidelines

gynaecology see women's health

H. pylori testing 246

haematology 297–8, 322

haematuria 322

handing over, consultation skills 93

'hard to reach' groups 148

headaches 273–4, 322
   see also neurological problems

health, WHO definition 107

health and safety 322

Health and Safety Executive 149, 170
health belief model 93, 138
health promotion 39, 107–9, 139, 322
    children and young people 190
    condensed know-how 167–9
    condensed knowledge 165–6
    condensed resources 170
    condensed skills 167
    men 211
    sexual health 219
Health Protection Agency (HPA) 113, 169
health surveillance 166, 169
    genetic conditions 174, 176
health visitors 322
    learning opportunities 28
    work with children and young people 192
healthcare services 166
Healthtalkonline 135
Healthy Child Programme, DH 194
Healthy Working UK website 234, 290, 291
hearing impairment 260
heart failure 322
hernias 322
heuristic teaching method 163
hidden curriculum 9
hidden presentation of illness 322
HIV (human immunodeficiency virus) 215, 217, 322
    prevention 219
holism, definition 117
holistic approach 39, 79, 117–18
home life, influence on care delivery 121
home oxygen therapy 281
home visits 322
Honey and Mumford's Learning Style Questionnaire 21
hormonal contraception 216
hospital posts 28–9
housekeeping
    in acute illness 182
    consultation skills 94
    end-of-life care 225
hypertension 322
hyperuricaemia 267
    condensed know-how 270–1
    condensed knowledge 267–9
hypothetico-deductive model 98

iatrogenic problems 289
IM&T (information management and technology) skills 39, 137, 144, 158
    respiratory health 280
imaging services 327
immunisation programmes 166, 168, 190, 322
    resources 170
immunisation for travel 327
Improving Access to Psychological Therapies programme 231
incidence of disease 98
inequalities in health provision 112, 322
infectious diseases 298–9, 322
infertility 322
influenza campaigns 322
informal curriculum 8
information sharing 149
informed consent 94
inheritance *see* genetics
Inner Consultation, The, Roger Neighbour 93–4
InnovAiT 134
intellectual disability 235
    condensed know-how 237–9
    condensed knowledge 235–6
    condensed skills 237
    condensed resources 239
interface management 88
International Planned Parenthood Foundation 222
International Society of Men's Health 213
interpersonal skills, Clinical Skills Assessment 51
inverse care law 112, 168
investigations 101, 322

Johari window 122
joint injections 286
joint surgeries 19, 84
journal watch services 33, 126
journals 33
justice 142

keeping up to date 33–4
King's Fund 112, 170
knowledge base 15–16
Knowledge Updates 33

language problems 50
leadership 86, 91, 152
    in emergencies 180
learning disabilities *see* intellectual
    disability
learner-centred approach 162
learning
    complex skills 26
    from experience 18–19
    feedback and formative
        assessment 30, 32
    keeping up to date 33–4
    from other health professionals
        28
    principles of 17–18
    problem-based 25
    reflective 19–20
    in secondary care 28–9
    self-awareness assessments 21
    self-directed 21–2
    by teaching 33
    tutorials 26
learning groups 27
learning log
    linking entries to curriculum
        areas 55
    preparation for Annual Review
        72
    writing high-quality entries 55,
        56
learning materials, curriculum
    statements 29–30
learning needs 22
    confidence rating 24
    identification 82–3
        by patient contact 24–5
        through educational activities
            23
learning outcomes 14, 15
    personal 26–7
learning portfolios 34–5
learning record 53
learning style preferences 21
learning tips 131–2
legal frameworks 120
life expectancies 112
lifestyle interventions 108
    metabolic problems 270
literature, critical appraisal 125–6
Liverpool Care Pathway 226
long-acting reversible contraception
    (LARC) 216, 219

lung cancer 281, 322

Macmillan Cancer Support 227
mailing lists, keeping up to date 34
major incidents 184
management plans 101
management structures 153
management theory and practice
    323
mandatory procedures 59–60
Marie Curie Cancer Care 226
maternity leave 323
MCQ *see* multiple-choice questions
medical records 106
    patient access 148
medical specialty placements 308–9
medically unexplained symptoms
    323
Medicines and Healthcare products
    Regulatory Agency 149
meeting of two experts consultation
    model 140
meetings 323
meningitis 323
men's health 208
    condensed know-how 211–12
    condensed knowledge 208–9
    condensed resources 213
    condensed skills 210
    three main themes 213
Men's Health Forum 213
menstrual disorders 201, 323
Mental Capacity Act 2005 239
mental health 228
    children and young people 194
    condensed know-how 231–3
    condensed knowledge 228–30
    condensed resources 233–4
    condensed skills 230–1
    older people 197
    women 201
Mental Health Act 1983 233, 234,
    323
mental health assessment skills, care
    of older people 195
mentoring 156, 159
metabolic problems 267
    condensed know-how 270–1
    condensed knowledge 267–9
    condensed resources 271–2
    condensed skills 269
methadone prescription 253

methotrexate 289
migraine 323
mini-clinical evaluation exercise
  (mini-CEX) 57, 58, 61
minor illnesses in adults 323
minor injuries 323
minor surgery 323
Misuse of Drugs Act 1971 253
mock CSAs 49
moles 323
moral reasoning 137
motivation 323
MRCGP assessment 37
    acronyms 42
    Annual Review of Competence
    Progression 72–3
    Applied Knowledge Test 43
        preparation 45–6
        question types 43–4
    Clinical Skills Assessment 46–7
        areas covered 48
        difference between passing
        and failing 50–2
        examples of cases 48
        marking 47
        preparation 47, 49–50
    competency areas 38, 39–40
    development 38
    relationship to the curriculum 40, 41
    Workplace-Based Assessment 52
        Annual Review of
        Competence Progression 70
        assessment side 52–3
        cardio-pulmonary
        resuscitation training 67
        case-based discussion 61–3
        Clinical Supervisor's Report
        68–9
        consultation observation tool
        63–4
        direct observation of
        procedural skills 59–60
        evidence collection 53–4
        evidence timetable 71
        final review 73
        importance 52
        learning side 53
        mini-clinical evaluation
        exercise 61
        multi-source feedback 66–7
        naturally occurring evidence
        54–5

out-of-hours experience 67–8
patient satisfaction
questionnaires 65
RCGP Trainee ePortfolio 53
six-monthly review 69–70
Workplace-Based Assessment
tools 55–9, 58
MRCGP examination 37
MSF see multi-source feedback
multidisciplinary team meetings 29
multidisciplinary working 123, 147
    with children and young people
    191
    metabolic problems 270
    musculoskeletal conditions 289
    respiratory health 281
    skin problems 295
multiple-choice questions, sample
    papers 46
multiple problems
    comprehensive approach 106–7
    prioritisation 85
multiple sclerosis 323
multi-source feedback (MSF) 58,
    66–7
musculoskeletal conditions 284
    condensed know-how 289–90
    condensed knowledge 284–7
    condensed resources 290–1
    condensed skills 288
    specialty-based placements
    312–13

narrative-based medicine 92
National Autistic Society 239
National Genetics Education and
    Development Centre 177
National Institute for Health and
    Clinical Excellence (NICE) 113,
    177
    clinical guidelines
        acute illnesses 185
        cardiovascular health 243
        children and young people
        193
        digestive health 249
        drug and alcohol misuse 254
        ENT problems 261
        eye problems 266
        genetic conditions 177
        men's health 213
        mental health 233

metabolic problems 271
musculoskeletal conditions 290
neurological problems 277
older people 199
referral for suspected cancer 227
respiratory conditions 282
sexual health 221
skin problems 296
women's health 207
practice guidelines 135
public health guidelines 170, 207, 221
drug and alcohol misuse 254
quality standards
alcohol dependence 254
chronic heart failure 243
COPD 282
diabetes 271
end-of-life care 226
stroke 277
National Osteoporosis Society 291
National Reporting and Learning Service 149
National Service Frameworks
for COPD 282
for coronary heart disease 244
for long-term conditions 277
for mental health 234
for older people 199
National Stroke Strategy 277
naturally occurring evidence 54–5
'navigator' role 115, 139
near-patient testing, DMARDs 287
neck lumps 323
needs-based learning 17–18
negotiation 91, 137
ENT problems 259
neonatal problems 190
neurological problems 273
condensed know-how 276–7
condensed knowledge 273–5
condensed resources 277
condensed skills 276
newborn genetic screening 176
Newborn Hearing Screening Programme 260
NHS Cancer Strategy for England 227
NHS Choices 135
NHS Evidence 135

NHS Quality Improvement Scotland (NHS QIS) 149
NHS structure 87, 112–13
non-attendance, children and young people 191
non-maleficence 142
non-medical agendas 114
notifiable diseases 166
nurse-led clinics, chronic disease management 242
nurse specialists
in diabetes mellitus 270
in ENT conditions 259
nurses, learning opportunities 28
nursing care 325

obesity 267, 324
condensed know-how 270–1
condensed knowledge 267–9
condensed resources 271–2
condensed skills 269
obstetrics 324
obstetrics and gynaecology placements 309
occupational health 169, 170, 299, 324
Healthy Working UK website 291
musculoskeletal conditions 290
occupational history 100
off legs 324
older adults, care of 195
condensed know-how 196–8
condensed resources 199
condensed skills 195
elderly care placements 305
on-call/on-take experience 303
ophthalmology placements 310
opiate misuse
symptoms 250
see also drug misuse
opportunity costs 109
optional procedures 60
oral contraception 324
organisational skills 90
osteoporosis 324
fracture risk assessment 285
see also musculoskeletal conditions
out-of-hours (OOH) care, organization 184
out-of-hours experience 67–8, 104, 178, 185

outpatient clinics 303
    learning opportunities 29

paediatric placements 310–11
paediatrics *see* children, care of
pain relief ladder 223
palliative care 324
    see also end-of-life care
Palliative Care Guidelines for
    Scotland 226
Palliative Care Matters website 226
palliative care placements 307
pancreatic cancer diagnosis 249
panel reviews 72
panic attacks 317
parents, support for 190
Parkinson's disease 324
partnership organization 324
partial sightedness 262, 265–6
partnership agreements 324
partnership with patients 95–7
patient advocate role 90
patient care pathways 88
patient-centred clinical method 140
Patient.co.uk 135
patient feedback 154
patient information leaflets 324
patient participation 324
patient safety and quality of care 143
    condensed know-how 145–9
    condensed resources 149
    condensed skills 143–5
patient satisfaction questionnaires
    (PSQ) 57, 58, 65
patients' objectives 160
peer study groups 34, 50
Pendleton feedback rules 32
pensions 324
performance maintenance 40
peripheral vascular disease 324
person-centred approach 48, 78,
    92–3, 110
    autonomy 94
    doctor–patient relationship 93–5
    management plans 101
    partnership with patients 95–7
personal continuity of care 96
Personal Development Plans (PDPs)
    22, 83
    preparation for Annual Review 72
    template 35
Personal Education Planning (PEP)

tools 24, 46
personal health 124
personal learning outcomes 26–7
personal life, influence on care
    delivery 121
pharmacists, learning opportunities
    28
PHQ-9 assessment 234
physiotherapists, learning
    opportunities 28
physiotherapy 324
Picker Institute 170
portfolios 34–5, 52–3
    RCGP Trainee ePortfolio 53–4
'postcode lotteries' 112
postnatal care 324
postnatal depression 205
poverty, impact on health 112
practical skills demonstration 48
practice finances 153, 324
practice managers 324
practice nurses 324
    learning opportunities 28
predictive values 105
pregnancy-related problems 201–2
premises 324
prescribing 158
    for children and young people
    190, 193
    for older people 196
prescribing monitoring 325
prescription charges exemption 271
prescriptions analysis 25
presentations 158
prevalence of disease 98
preventive activities 83, 107–9, 166,
    325
    children and young people 189
    digestive health 247
    genetic conditions 174
    HIV prevention 219
    men's health 211
    metabolic problems 269
    musculoskeletal health 287
    older people 198
    respiratory health 280
    sexual health 217
    skin problems 294
    women's health 203
primary care administration 39
Primary Care Dermatology Society
    296

Primary Care Genetics Society 177
primary care management 48, 78
   chronic disease management
    81–2
   communication skills 86, 89
   consultation skills 81
   'gatekeeper' role 91
   identification of learning needs
    82–3
   interface management 88
   knowledge of NHS structure 87
   knowledge of Primary Care
    Organisation 86
   organisational skills 90
   patient advocate role 90
   preventive activities 83
   prioritisation of problems 85
   referral processes 88
   service management and service
    improvement 89
   skill development 83–4
    clinical skills 84
    therapeutic skills 84–5
   team working and leadership
    86–7
   understanding epidemiology of
    primary care problems 80–1
Primary Care Organisation 86
Primary Care Respiratory Society
  283
Primary Care Rheumatology
  Society 291
primary care team 153
prioritisation of problems 85
problem-based approach 100
problem-based learning 18, 25–6
problem case analysis 24
problem-solving skills 48, 78, 98–9,
  325
   urgent intervention 103–4
   use of information 100–1
   working principles 102–3
procedural skills, DOPS 59–60
procedures, in acute illness 181
professional boundaries 95
Programme Directors 6
prostate disorders 325
protocols 325
PSQ *see* patient satisfaction
  questionnaires
psychiatric emergencies 325
psychiatric placements 311–12

psychological distress, ENT
  symptoms 260
psychological therapies 231
psychosexual counselling 222
psychosexual problems 325
psychosocial issues
  metabolic disease 271
  skin problems 296
  women's health 206
psychosomatic complaints 232
public health 113
public health professionals 168, 170
PUNs & DENs 24

QRISK 2-2012 calculator 244
quality assurance 114, 143, 325
quality improvement 147–9
Quality and Outcomes Framework
  (QOF) 114
question sources, Applied
  Knowledge Test 45
question types, Applied Knowledge
  Test 43–4

random case analysis 25
rapport 95
rationing of resources 115
RCGP Essential Knowledge
  Challenges 46
RCGP online courses
  alcohol- and drug-related issues
   254
  domestic violence 207
  mental health 234
  musculoskeletal conditions 291
  pancreatic cancer diagnosis 249
  respiratory health 283
  sexual health 221
RCGP Substance Misuse and
  Associated Health unit 254
RCGP Trainee ePortfolio 53
  evidence collection 53–4
   naturally occurring evidence
    54–5
   writing learning log entries
    55, 56
  templates 54
  Workplace-Based Assessment
   tools 55–9, 58
recessive single-gene disorders 173
record keeping 90, 325
  medical records 106

red eye 325
red flags 104
    digestive health 248
    ENT conditions 260
    musculoskeletal conditions 284
    in older people 196
referral 88, 139, 325
    cardiovascular services 242
    for ENT conditions 259
    genetic conditions 176
    metabolic problems 270
    musculoskeletal conditions 289
    sexual health services 219
    skin problems 295, 296
    for suspected cancer 227
    women's health 205
referrals analysis 25
reflective diaries 123
reflective learning 17, 19–20
    learning portfolios 35
reflective practice 122, 137, 143
    drug and alcohol misuse 252
    end-of-life care 225
    mental health 231
    sexual health 218
reflux 321
regulatory frameworks 120
Relate 222
relationship difficulties 325
relationships with colleagues 325
relationships with patients 325
renal problems 298, 325
repeat prescriptions 325
research 325
research methodologies 157
research placements 312
research skills 159, 161
residential care 325
resource allocation 148
resource management 138
resources 135
    RCGP curriculum 134
respiratory health 278
    condensed know-how 281–2
    condensed knowledge 278–80
    condensed resources 282–3
    condensed skills 280
responsibility 139
resuscitation 325
resuscitation guidelines 182, 185
resuscitation training 67, 104
revalidation 114

role of the curriculum 3
Revalidation ePortfolio 34–5
revision courses 49
rheumatology placements 312–13
risk assessment 143, 145–6
    drug and alcohol misuse 252
risk calculators 99
risk factors 165, 169
risk management
    in acute illness 182
    men's issues 210
role models 7, 9
role-play 49
Rome III criteria 246
routine health checks 242

safety of patients see patient safety
    and quality of care
safety-netting 93, 102, 181
SBA see single best answer questions
scientific features 119, 125–6
Scottish Intercollegiate Guidelines
    Network (SIGN) 135
screening 166, 168, 318, 326
    antenatal and newborn 176
    for colorectal cancer 248
    for COPD 281
    for eye problems 265
    men's health 211
    newborn hearing screening 260
    resources 170
    sexual health 220
    for Type 2 diabetes 270
    Wilson and Junger criteria 171
    women's health 205, 207
secondary care interactions 88
secondary care learning 28–9
secondary care referrals 88
Self Care Forum 290
self-awareness 122, 123, 152
    drug and alcohol misuse 252
    mental health 231
    sexual health 218
self-awareness assessments 21
self-directed learning 17, 21–2
self-harm, deliberate 326
self-management, patients 124, 160
    ENT conditions 260
    metabolic conditions 271
    musculoskeletal conditions 290
    respiratory conditions 280, 281
serious illness, recognition 29

service development 152
service management and service
   improvement 89, 113–14, 123–4
service organisation 153–4
seven-tasks consultation model 140
sexual dysfunction 219
sexual health 214, 321
   condensed know-how 218–21
   condensed knowledge 214–17
   condensed resources 221–2
   condensed skills 217–18
sexual health medicine placements
   308
sexual history-taking 218
shared care, metabolic problems 270
shared surgeries 49
sickness certification 326
SIGN guidelines
   acute illnesses 185
   cardiovascular health 243
   children and young people 193
   dementia 199
   digestive health 249
   drug and alcohol misuse 254
   ENT problems 261
   men's health 213
   mental health 233
   metabolic problems 271
   musculoskeletal conditions 290
   neurological problems 277
   respiratory conditions 282
   sexual health 221
   skin problems 296
   women's health 207
Significant Event Analysis (SEA)
   146–7, 326
Single Assessment Process (SAP)
   111
single best answer questions (SBA)
   44
six-monthly review 69–70
skill development 83–5
skills simulator laboratories 50
skin problems 292
   condensed know-how 295–6
   condensed knowledge 292–4
   condensed resources 296
   condensed skills 294–5
smoking 326
   attitudes towards 281, 282
smoking cessation 280
social care, interrelationships with

health care 111
social history 100
social responsibilities 155
socioeconomic factors
   impact on health 112
   in mental health 232–3
Socratic teaching method 163
specialty-based placements 303–13
spiral learning 8, 31
sports injuries 326
staff development skills 151
stages of a consultation 140
Standards for Better Health Care,
   seven domains 150
statement sections 11
statements
   guardians 5
   initial development 4
statistics 156, 159, 326
sterilisation 326
steroids, topical 293
stroke 326
   condensed resources 277
   RCP guidelines 244
   see also neurological problems
subjectivity, doctor–patient
   relationship 95
Subutex prescription 253
suicide 326
summarising, consultation skills 93
summative assessment 37–8
superannuation 324
supervision 41–2, 156
support services, older people 197
surgery 299, 326

table completion questions 44
teaching 156, 159, 162
   learning by 33
teaching methods 163
teaching skills 326
teaching tips 131–2
team working 39, 86–7, 110, 137,
   144, 147, 151–2
   respiratory health 281
   sexual health services 219
technical skills log 53
teenage health care 326
Teenage Pregnancy Strategy 221
telephone consultations 326
templates, ePortfolio 54
terminal illness see end-of-life care

termination of pregnancy 206, 216, 326
Terrence Higgins Trust 222
thyroid disorders 267, 326
  condensed know-how 270–1
  condensed knowledge 267–9
  condensed skills 269
time, as a diagnostic tool 102, 327
time management 326
tolerance 118
topical steroids 293
Trainee ePortfolio 34
trainees, value of the curriculum 3
training difficulties, use of the curriculum 30, 31
Training Record 53
transference 123
travel advice 327
treatment decisions 84–5
tutorials 26

UK Vision Strategy 266
uncertainty 102–3, 320, 327
Unique 177
updating courses 126
urgent intervention 103–4
  dangerous diagnoses 186
  see also acute illness
urinary tract problems 298, 327

venous thrombosis 327
vertigo 327
video consultations 18–19, 49, 64
violence 327
visual impairment 262, 265–6, 327
vomiting 320
vulnerable groups 148

warfarin monitoring 327
Whooley questions 229
Women's health 200
  condensed know-how 205–6
  condensed knowledge 200–3
  condensed resources 207
  condensed skills 204
  obstetrics and gynaecology placements 309–10
work, relationship to health 169
work–life balance 97, 124, 327
working environment, influence on care delivery 121
working principles 102–3

workload, influence on care delivery 120
Workplace-Based Assessment (WPBA) 38, 52
  Annual Review of Competence Progression 70, 72–3
  assessment side 52–3
  cardio-pulmonary resuscitation training 67
  case-based discussion 61–3
  Clinical Supervisor's Report 68–9
  competency areas 38, 39–40
  consultation observation tool 63–4
  direct observation of procedural skills 59–60
  evidence collection 53–4
    naturally occurring evidence 54–5
    writing learning log entries 55, 56
  evidence timetable 71
  final review 73
  importance 52
  learning side 53
  mini-clinical evaluation exercise 61
  multi-source feedback 66–7
  out-of-hours experience 67–8
  patient satisfaction questionnaires 65
  RCGP Trainee ePortfolio 53
  six-monthly review 69–70
Workplace-Based Assessment tools 30, 55–9, 58
  multi-source feedback 58
  optional tools 59
  tools used in primary care 57
  tools used in secondary care 57

X-linked single-gene disorders 173
X-rays 327

yellow flags, musculoskeletal conditions 289
young people, care of 187
  condensed know-how 190–3
  condensed knowledge 187–9
  condensed resources 193–4
  condensed skills 189
  contraception and sexual health 220

mental health 232
musculoskeletal conditions 286
paediatric placements 310–11
visual impairment 265